Dental Documentation
With Confidence

The "Go-To" Documentation Guide for the Clinical Team

Stay in Compliance and Maximize Legitimate Reimbursement

2023 EDITION

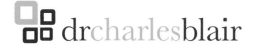
drcharlesblair

704.829.3194 / practicebooster.com

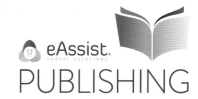
eAssist
PUBLISHING

Register your 2023 Edition

Book Registration / Dental Documentation With Confidence

Name:
_____

Address:
_____

_____

Telephone: _____   Email _____

Fax to: 704.825.3960

Email or scan to: info@practicebooster.com

Mail to: Practice Booster, P.O. BOX 986, Belmont, NC 28012

Thank you for registering!

Comments

If you would like to provide a testimonial or suggestion, or if you find an error in this guide, please complete the form below:

Name:
_____

Address:
_____

_____

Telephone: _____   Email: _____

Please check one of the following:

◯ Testimonial   ◯ Suggestion   ◯ Error (Please indicate the code and page number.)

Comments:
_____

_____

_____

_____

Fax to: 704.825.3960

Email or scan to: info@practicebooster.com

Thank you for your contribution!

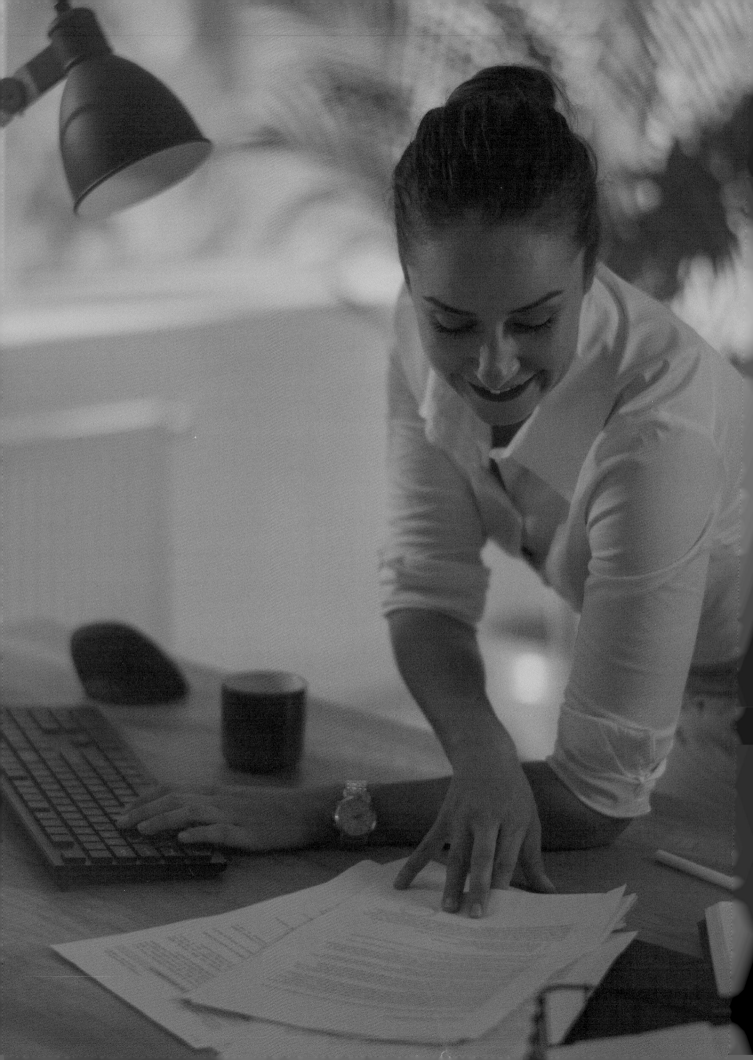

Table of Contents

Documentation is the cornerstone
for keeping you in compliance and
maximizing legitimate reimbursement.

Introduction

Documentation is the cornerstone for keeping you in compliance and maximizing legitimate reimbursement. So much so, that we have created this book as a way for you to access everything you need to know when it comes to obtaining and recording proper documentation. There is so much to know and remembering every single detail is not always realistic. Whether you are new to dentistry or a seasoned member of the dental community, this book will serve you in more ways than you can count. With this tool in your toolbox, you will be able to document with confidence and focus on what you do best, building trusting and lasting relationships with your patients and providing the quality of care they deserve.

The saying of "you cannot document enough" is an understatement and is something we emphasize when teaching the importance of taking good chart notes.

The Why of Documentation

The Consequences of Improper Documentation

The need to properly document a patient's clinical findings has certainly evolved over the last 100 years. Federal regulations, technology, and the legal aspect of what we do have forced us to be thorough when documenting. The saying of "you cannot document enough" is an understatement and is something we emphasize when teaching the importance of taking good chart notes.

As the need for record keeping has evolved, so has the need for intaking and evaluating a patient's health history. This has truly become a key component of all dental treatment and can not be overlooked when documenting. Some patients do not see us as medical professionals; thus, stressing to the patient the importance of thorough and accurate health information is vital to the documentation process. Helping them understand their oral health is systemic and impactful to their overall health is something we all must do to help the patient truly understand their current health status as well as for ensuring we are documenting medical necessity for treatment rendered.

Dental records contain sensitive information; personal information including a patient's name, date of birth and social security number, insurance information such as the employer, policy name, group plan or member identification number, and of course clinical information such as current findings, diagnosis of treatment needed, as well as radiographs and intraoral images to support the diagnosis.

Obtaining financial reimbursements from insurance on behalf of the patient requires accurate recording of findings, diagnosis, and treatment precisely. This provides a detailed description of not only why treatment was rendered, but how treatment was provided for optimal health of the patient. Radiographs and intraoral images become invaluable tools when needing to provide supporting documentation for a narrative or appeal for payment.

While the dentist collects the needed information from the patient and stores it for them, the records actually belong to the patient and may be requested at any time. With the advent of technology, sharing that information has become easier and more efficient. Keeping quality and detailed records ensures the dental practice has done their due diligence of keeping patients informed and educated.

In 1996, the Health Insurance Portability and Accountability Act (HIPAA) was signed into law and has impacted the way we create and store patient records. It promotes the security and privacy of patient information including how and who we share it. Violations and fines can run into the hundreds of thousands of dollars and affect every member of the healthcare team. Annual training is required to ensure the privacy and security of patients' healthcare information; documenting training has been completed is just as important as any other information we collect.

The passage of the 21st Century Cures Act solidifies patients' rights by allowing unrestrained access to their electronic health information which is updated automatically, in a way that is easy to understand, and is secure. Patients must be given immediate access to their records upon request, no exceptions.

At any time, these records can be called into evidence by a dental board or a court of law. This realization of documenting "evidence" crystalizes the necessity of being as thorough as we can when recording information. When chart notes are created, the thought of this information being called on one day as legal documentation is not always at the forefront of our minds. Hence, the imperative of documenting properly each and every time. Done correctly, documentation will be the provider's biggest asset. Done incorrectly, it may be their largest liability. If the practice is audited, summoned for peer or dental board review, or is faced with legal action, there is nothing more valuable than thorough and legible chart notes. Technically, if it is not documented, it did not happen. If it is written down, but no one can read it, it still did not happen. Making the importance of signing and dating what procedures, symptoms, etc. extremely critical.

Clinical Record Documentation

When under state dental board or peer review, it is important the clinical record supports the information reported on the claim form. If it is not in the chart, it did not legally happen. The clinical record should contain the patient's chief complaint (if applicable) or reason for the visit, the diagnosis prior to treatment, related radiographs and photos of the area of the oral cavity and/or tooth to help establish the need for treatment, the type, amount, and method of delivery for any anesthesia, the treatment provided with as much detail as possible, prescriptions and instructions given, the initials or signature of the treating providers, date, and any other relevant information.

Remember, there are three recommendations to help circumvent negative results from any type of review or audit: document, document, document! These same principals hold true for properly maintaining clinical records and submitting claims on a regular basis.

When recording chart notes, they must be clear and concise, not containing "slang", office lingo, or uncommon abbreviations. If chart notes are hand written, they must be legible. In any situation, if the insurance company, the dental board, or a court of law can not read or understand the notes, they will be dismissed and not used to determine reimbursement or determine liability.

It is important to stick to the facts of the visit and record what the patient is telling you; descriptions or symptoms or a reference they make when talking to you. Document visual assessments such as swelling, redness, an open sore, etc. Be professional in the assessment and be sure to document any complications that occur while providing treatment. Also, ensure you are documenting vital signs as part of a thorough health screening.

Ideally, thorough clinical record documentation contains periodontal charting completed annually to track bone loss and determine the need for treatment. When seeking reimbursement for any type of periodontal necessity, this charting becomes invaluable.

Notes

Every chart entry must be signed
and dated by the doctor or associate
provider rendering treatment.

CHAPTER TWO

Proper Documentation

Elements of Proper Chart Notes

The importance of complete and legible chart notes has been established. Now, let us review the essential elements of a chart note. Every chart entry must be signed and dated by the doctor or associate provider rendering treatment. In addition, any team member(s) assisting the doctor or hygienist in treating the patient should also be listed in the chart note. If the treatment is provided by someone other than the doctor, this person should write the chart note, sign, and date it. The doctor will then need to review the chart note, sign, and date as well. This proves the doctor is aware of all treatment provided to the patient.

Additionally, there should be as much continuity and standardization between all doctors and team members in the office as possible. The use of common dental abbreviations is allowed. However, since abbreviations will vary slightly from one practice to another, abbreviation meanings need to be consistent in every record. Provide a "key" to the abbreviations used in the practice to ensure all team members utilize the same abbreviations and understand what they mean, so anyone writing or reading a record is familiar with what is being conveyed. The abbreviation "key" should be placed in all operatories, for easy access. Be certain all patient records contain consistent and accurate information. This key will help all team members (past, present, and future) function appropriately in maintaining the legal record.

Paper chart notes must be free from scribbles and whiteout errors. If errors are made, draw a thin single line through the error (in ink pen), date and initial, and add the correction. Notations should be written without blank lines or large spaces between the entries. This prevents notes from being added at a later time.

Corrections in computerized formats will vary according to the dental software. Most will "lock" the data and will only allow amendments. These amendments should contain any additional information or corrections with a notation marking them as a revision or correction and refer back to the original note.

Chart Notes Should Include (but are not limited to):

- Date and description of evaluation

- Reason for ordering radiographs and which radiographs are requested

- Reason for ordering intraoral or extraoral 2D photographic images and which images are requested

- A notation stating the radiographs or images were reviewed by the provider

- Date and description of all radiographs, diagnostic casts (study models), and periodontal charting

- Date and description of treatment or services rendered

- Date and description of treatment complications

- Date, name of, quantity of, and strength of all drugs dispensed, administered, or prescribed and refills (if applicable)

- Diagnosis – in addition to an overall diagnosis (e.g., rampant caries, generalized moderate periodontitis), each tooth requiring treatment should also have a diagnosis

- Record of lab results

- Record of health history and health history updates

- Record of every canceled or missed appointment

- Record of patient accepting or refusing treatment

- Record of all pertinent discussions/communication with the patient whether in person, by phone, letter, email, text, or internet video or audio call

- Record of all referrals and explanation for the referral

- Record of all consultations with the patient's physician

- Recommendation for treatment at the next visit (treatment plan)

Never include negative, disparaging, or personal judgments regarding the patient, as this is not objective and lessens professional credibility. Choose language which documents what happened without insult, such as saying "pt. chose not to proceed with" instead of "pt. refused". Do not use internal abbreviations to communicate that a patient is 'difficult.' Keep it professional and clinical. Remember, patients can access their records at any point and may be reading the chart themselves.

Far too many practices face disciplinary or malpractice action due to poorly documented patient records. This fact is both disappointing and surprising, especially since today's technology makes it very easy to create appropriate chart notes. Sadly, failure to properly document causes problems not only for doctors, but for their patients. When a patient transfers to a new doctor, a poorly documented chart may fail to provide adequate

information for the new provider to be fully educated on the patient's medical and dental history, including when and why previous treatment was performed. These facts are vital should a claim arise for replacing these restorations. Since chart notes also serve to inform the doctor, clinical, and administrative team of what treatment is planned (and in what order), as well as provide a record of what treatment was completed and why, lacking or illegible chart notes can cause needless confusion.

Most dental practices are equipped with current computer technology. Today's dental practice management software systems make it easy to properly document dental services chairside during the oral evaluation and treatment appointments by the doctor, dental assistant, or hygienist. Computerized workstations in operatories allow the dental team to document all necessary information directly into the patient's electronic chart. Even if the practice is not computerized, it is still critical that all chart notes are recorded legibly and in detail **at the time of service** to ensure the information charted is complete and accurate. All too often, this information is charted after the fact and important details are missed or forgotten unintentionally, and consequently left undocumented.

Electronic protected health information (ePHI) must meet HIPAA standards, so confidentiality remains a chief concern with software systems. Clear steps must be taken to ensure that patient information is neither shared nor accessible to unauthorized parties. Furthermore, the authenticity of the original record must be maintained with any electronic transmissions, so the practice must ensure its dental software system offers both confidentiality and the ability to retain the integrity of the original records. Keep in mind when selecting a computerized charting program that the inability to change entries at a later date must be part of the program. After an entry is entered and signed, the only way to change the entry should be to amend it by adding a new chart note; once entered, an existing entry must be inalterable.

Thorough and Accurate
Chart Notes Allow:

1. The doctor and dental assistant reviewing the diagnosis to identify what treatment was previously performed and what treatment is needed next

2. The hygienist(s) reviewing the diagnosis to identify what treatment the doctor has recommended and when it is time to schedule recare appointments

3. The front office team to easily determine what services should be billed to the patient and what to submit to the patient's insurance payor

4. The coroner to see proper records and notes for identification purposes in the event of the patient's death

5. The insurance company to see all required records and notes that will be scrutinized if an audit is performed

6. Patient records to be transferred to a peer review committee or a State Dental Board for whom records are critical should there be questions about treatment

7. Attorneys and juries to have thorough and accurate chart notes, which is the best defense in the event of a lawsuit

If the practice is audited, summoned for peer or dental board review, or is faced with legal action, there is nothing more valuable than thorough and legible chart notes. ∎

Notes

Obtaining and documenting a
thorough dental history is essential
to maintaining proper patient records.

Documenting Medical and Dental History

3

Medical histories have become the true foundation for all dental treatment. We understand the oral systemic connection all too well now and realize the importance of maintaining good oral health in order to maintain proper physical health.

Our patients however, do not always understand this and therefore, do not realize the importance of accurate and up-to-date medical histories. We are healthcare providers, and as such, it is our job to educate patients on this very important piece of information before treatment is rendered. Patients often question why they need to update this information at each visit, yet the truth is, they do it every time they go into their medical doctor's office, so why not with us?

Documenting Medical Histories

When documenting medical history it is important to review every aspect of a patient's written form to ensure we understand it. Often times, they will leave out information due to a lack of understanding its applicability.

Scenario: A patient was seen in a dental office but did not feel the need to disclose the fact they had a Pacemaker placed just prior to the dental appointment. The patient had a tooth which had broken off and required a crown. Upon diagnosis and treatment acceptance, the patient was anesthetized with Epinephrine. During the procedure, the patient expressed concerns about a rapid heart beat. The doctor reassured the patient

this was very common with anesthesia, to take a couple of deep breaths and the feeling should go away. The patient then asked, "Will this affect my Pace-maker?" The doctor looked at the health history only to find there was no mention of a Pacemaker, which prompted the doctor to ask, "I see you updated your health history today yet made no mention of this; how long have you had that?" The patient replied, "Three weeks, did you need to know that?"

The above scenario is one reason why the medical history for each patient should be updated at each visit, regardless of how far apart the appointments are. Asking questions that are open ended like, "When was the last time you were seen in the emergency room?" will get you more information than what has been disclosed on the medical form. "Oh, the last time I went to the ER was because of heart palpitations" or "I had a reaction to medication I was given".

Another question to ask is, "When was the last time your doctor changed your medication?" You will find that many times, in recalling when a medication had been changed, they will give you a different medication than what is written down from previous visits. Reviewing the medical history, at length, will paint a more accurate picture of your patient's health as it relates to dentistry.

Patients should be required to **_sign and date_** their medical and dental history updates. Their signature acts as an acknowledgment that these have been reviewed with them in depth and that what is documented is true and accurate. Without a signature, it is your word against theirs. Obtaining their signature and date is validation for everyone that all are well informed. If, for whatever reason, the patient has chosen **not** to disclose something, their signature solidifies that as well!

Obtaining and documenting a thorough dental history is essential to maintaining proper patient records. A patient's dental history helps support the rendering provider's clinical assessment, aids in determining an accurate diagnosis, and helps develop a comprehensive preventive and therapeutic treatment plan for each patient.

In order to record the patient's dental history, the dentist and/or staff member(s) should obtain a complete and thorough dental history from the patient. Note any information offered by the patient about current fears and concerns, as well as any details shared about past dental experiences.

The patient's oral health conditions, as observed on the day of the evaluation, should also be recorded. The clinical observations that should be recorded in the patient's dental history include, but are not limited to: previous restorations, periodontal treatment, extractions, orthodontic treatment, oral habits, and patient reactions to treatment, including anesthesia experiences and the efficacy of the anesthesia methods. Additionally, intraoral photographs should be taken for a baseline comparison.

It is important the names of previous dentists are obtained and the appropriate record releases are signed by the patient or custodial individual prior to the patient's initial visit. This allows any past patient documentation or records to be requested and obtained from prior treating providers, as deemed necessary by the current treating dentist, prior to the patient's evaluation. Having the necessary documentation from the previous dentist(s) in hand at the initial evaluation visit can greatly enhance the dentist's ability to complete the initial evaluation process without having to wait for the supportive historical information.

What Does a Dental History Include?

There is some basic information which is essential to include in the patient's dental history. In addition, it is also helpful to determine the patient's overall caries risk. Let us look at what elements a dental history should include for a child patient, for example.

According to the American Academy of Pediatric Dentistry (AAPD), a dental history on a child should address the following:

- Chief complaint.
- Previous dental experience.
- Date of last dental visit.
- Date of last radiographs.
- Oral hygiene habits and practices.
- Fluoride use/exposure history.
- Dietary habits (including bottle/ no-spill training cup use in young children).
- Sports activities.
- Previous orofacial trauma.
- Temporomandibular joint (TMJ) history.
- Family history of caries.
- Social development.

In addition to recording the patient's past experiences, noting the caries risk factors, and determining the caries risk level, the condition of the patient's oral cavity should also be documented at the first appointment.

Today, many dental practices utilize technology to streamline this documentation process. Technology used by dental teams may include an intraoral camera, CariVuTM, radiographic images, cone beam computed tomography (CBCT), and/or voice recordings. By utilizing some or all of these

3

technologies and techniques, the process of recording the present dental conditions is augmented and the time, energy, and efforts needed are reduced.

The images captured by an intraoral camera are an exact representation of the existing condition of the patient's mouth. On the other hand, a "drawing" or computer generated "free hand" tooth chart of existing restorations and conditions is not as accurate nor as graphic as photographic and radiographic images. With proper training, the images captured by an intraoral camera improve accuracy and reduce the time needed to record the existing conditions found in the mouth when the patient presents for an evaluation. Whether or not the practice utilizes these technologies or chooses to create manual documentation, charting of the existing conditions, restorations, and anatomy should be included in the clinical record.

Risk Factors to Note for Children 0-5 Years Old

Biological:

- Does the parent or primary caregiver have active caries?

- What is the parent or primary caregiver's socioeconomic status?

- How many sugar-containing snacks or beverages does the child consume per day (between meals)? (More or less than three?)

- Does the child have special care needs?

- Is the child a recent immigrant?

Protective:

- Does the child receive optimally fluoridated drinking water or fluoride supplements?

- Does the child brush his teeth daily with fluoridated toothpaste?

- Does the child receive topical fluoride from a health professional?

- Does the child have a "dental home" or receive regular dental care?

Clinical Findings:

- How many decayed/missing/filled surfaces does the child have?

- Does the child have active white spot lesions or enamel defects?

- Does the child have elevated mutans streptococci levels?

- Does the child have plaque on his/her teeth?

Risk Factors to Note for Children 6 and Older

Biological:

- Is the patient low socioeconomic status?

- How many sugar-containing snacks or beverages does the patient consume per day (between meals)? (More or less than three?)

- Is the child put to bed with a bottle containing natural or added sugar?

- Does the patient have special health care needs?

- Is the patient a recent immigrant?

Protective:

- Does the patient receive optimally fluoridated drinking water?

- Does the patient brush their teeth daily with fluoridated toothpaste?

- Has the patient received topical fluoride from a health professional?

- Does the patient use additional home measures (e.g., xylitol, MI paste, antimicrobial)?

- Does the patient have a "dental home" or receive regular dental care?

Clinical Findings:

- How many interproximal lesions does the patient have?

- Does the patient have active white spot lesions or enamel defects?

- Does the patient have low salivary flow?

- Does the patient have defective restorations?

- Is the patient wearing an intraoral appliance?

Once the caries risk factors are determined and an assessment is made (using recognized assessment tools), the overall caries risk for the patient can be determined and recorded. Recognized assessment tools are available from the ADA, California Dental Association, and AAPD.

Once a baseline dental history is obtained from the patient, the information should be recorded either electronically or using a pre-developed comprehensive dental history form. The patient or caregiver should sign the dental history form, confirming the information shared verbally with the dentist or qualified dental staff member is complete and accurate. This form should never be altered and should be kept in the clinical notes as a reference to previous treatments and the patient's recollection of those treatments, as well as any other contributing factors. Manual forms should be scanned into the patient's clinical record or included in a paper record.

It is vital to obtain a complete dental history and to properly record it in the patient's clinical record. This dental history can be used to help support the provider's clinical assessment. It can also help determine an accurate diagnosis and help develop a comprehensive preventive and therapeutic treatment plan tailored for each patient. Failing to obtain and record the dental history for each patient may hinder the dentist's ability to provide quality care for patients.

Telephone calls

All telephone calls regarding patient care should be entered into the patient record based on accurate and objective notes taken by the team member during the actual conversation. Best practice is to enter these notes into the patient record as soon as possible so they are not misplaced or forgotten. The patient, parent, or legal guardian must be verified and addressed directly. Quotation marks (" ") should be used anytime an actual conversation is being documented. When speaking with the guardian, legal representative, physician or insurance representative, also identify by name the person being quoted. Documentation of any conversations regarding financial matters need to be entered in the patient's financial record, not their clinical record. As a final reminder, in order to maintain privacy, always hold telephone conversations out of earshot of other patients.

Notes

The SOAP method is a great way to ensure all elements of proper chart notes are included.

CHAPTER FOUR

SOAP Note and PARQ Methods

A common method of documentation employed by many healthcare providers is using the SOAP method, which is an acronym for subjective, objective, assessment, and plan. This is a great way to ensure all elements of proper chart notes are included. The four components of a SOAP note are:

Subjective

A brief statement of the patient's purpose for the office visit or a description, location, and duration of symptoms quoted in the patient's own words. This is also known as the chief complaint and includes reviewing/updating medical history. These are things the patient tells you.

Assessment

The diagnosis(ses) of the patient's condition based upon subjective and objective findings.

S O A P

Objective

Unbiased observations by the doctor and dental team members which include the patient's vital signs (blood pressure, pulse, respiration) and any results of examinations (e.g., perio readings, what is seen on any radiographs taken, etc.). Basically, the facts that can be seen, heard, felt, measured, touched, and smelled.

Plan

The proposed, unique, treatment plan addressing the patient's problem(s). Be specific. For example, "caries" is too general of a diagnosis. Instead, each separate tooth (as well as each surface on each tooth) that is carious should be listed. This should also include the discussion with the patient regarding their condition as well as their decision regarding treatment (i.e., when the patient plans to proceed with treatment, if the patient has been referred to another provider for treatment, or if the patient has declined treatment).

Informed Consent

Informed consent must be obtained from the patient prior to providing treatment. Informed consent means the patient was fully informed of the treatment to be performed (both pros and cons), was allowed to ask questions, and the patient is of legal age and of sound mind. Patients may provide informed consent verbally (implied) or in writing. In the case of a lawsuit, implied consent is much less reliable, making written, signed consent preferable. Patients also have the right to refuse treatment in which case the provider should obtain a signed informed refusal from the patient.

If treatment changes during delivery, such as a filling turning into a root canal and crown, the procedure should be halted, the patient informed, and consent obtained before continuing with treatment. The potential for such changes should be discussed prior to treatment being initiated if changes are suspected or likely to occur.

The PARQ system is widely used in dentistry to ensure proper treatment plan discussions with the patient. This formula is extremely helpful:

Procedure
Describe recommended procedures/treatment plan to patient.

Alternatives
Describe any alternatives to the recommended treatment (including refusal of treatment). Also explain the possible outcome if treatment is rendered.

Risks
Explain any risks that may be involved with proceeding with treatment, as well as the risks of declining treatment.

Questions
Allow the patient to ask any questions and answer all questions thoroughly.

SOAP/PARQ Example:

Date: 11/07/2021

S — Patient indicated, "My top gum is swollen" and points to #3 and says, "My mouth tastes bad and it bleeds when I brush in that area."

O — Reviewed health hx: perio readings #3 WNL (within normal limits) except MF is 6mm and ML is 5mm, ML bleeding and buccal furcation exudate present after probing; requested PA and BW of #3 due to clinical evidence of pathology; PA & BW show approx 3mm bone loss on mesial, no caries, no PA radiolucency.

A — Periodontal abscess #3.

P and PARQ — Procedure explained; alternatives explained – tx by curetting the pocket or do not treat, pt chose treatment; risks explained, all pt questions were answered; 2% xylo w/ 1/100,000 epi 1.8 ml; curetted mesial #3; gave post-op instructions – warm saline rinse q4h, while awake, for 24 hr, OHI given; next visit: comp perio eval; JDoctor, DMD assisted by SMiles.

Informed Consent – Group Practices

Doctors in group practices must be aware that consent for one doctor to perform treatment is not consent for another doctor to perform the same treatment unless the patient has agreed to this. When applicable, the doctor performing the treatment must make an entry into the chart that the patient has agreed to the change of the treating doctor.

Amending Chart Notes

Never alter or add to original chart notes after the fact. However, chart notes may be amended if an error is noted or if something was mistakenly omitted. In this scenario, be sure to also date and sign the amended chart note(s).

Amended Chart Note Example:

Date: 11/09/2019

S — Patient indicates, "My tooth is sensitive to sweets" and points to #2.

O — Pt new to practice, came in on emergency basis; rev. health hx; visual exam shows #2 occlusal caries, requested BW due to carious lesion, BW shows #2 mesial caries; perio readings WNL on #2.

A — Mesial occlusal caries on #3.

P and **PARQ** — Recommended MO restoration; alternatives of gold inlay, ceramic inlay, MO amalgam, MO composite and tx explained, pt chose MO amal, risks explained of each alternative, pt questions answered; 2% xylo w/ 1/100,000 epi 1.8 ml; removed caries, placed MO amalgam.
Told patient to follow a soft diet for 24 hours and to call if sensitivity persists. Next visit: comp oral eval and FMX VHunter, DMD assisted by DIreland.

11-9-2019 Error in transcription. Assessment: on 11-9-19 note should have indicated mesial occlusal caries on #2 VHunter, DMD.

Some practices utilizing paper charts will draw a line through the incorrect part of a chart note, and attempt to write in the correction over it. However, this method is not recommended since maintaining legibility is critical. This process may make the entry too difficult to read (not only the initial error but also the correction). Rather, simply create a new chart entry, as outlined above, to correct any chart note errors.

The patient's chart should contain a diagnosis for each tooth that requires treatment. For example:

- **#18** – Current MOD amalgam, caries around amalgam and caries on buccal near the gingiva, DL cusp fractured off

- **#19** – In crossbite, no existing restoration, but patient complains of pain when eating, Tooth Slooth® is positive for fracture into dentin on ML and DL cusps

- **#27** – 3mm gingival recession on facial, 1mm attached gingiva

- **#29** – Existing crown placed 2004, caries on facial and distal at crown margin

- **#30** – Missing, extracted 2008

- **#31** – No existing restoration, deep caries on mesial and occlusal, but pulp tests normal and patient does not complain of sensitivity

The entries above, along with a full series of radiographs and a complete periodontal charting would provide adequate narrative/documentation to submit the following treatment plan:

- **#18** Crown
- **#19** Crown
- **#27** Subepithelial connective tissue graft procedure
- **#29** Retainer crown
- **#30** Pontic
- **#31** Retainer crown

Excellent chart notes include a diagnosis for treatment recommended on each tooth, which allows team members to copy the diagnosis for submission of the narrative (note, the doctor should review the narrative reported on all claims). 📶

Notes

CHAPTER FIVE

The Importance of Images

A picture is worth a thousand words

Many patients are expressing heightened awareness and concern regarding the taking of dental radiographs due to widespread internet access and media attention regarding potential harmful effects of radiation. Justified or not, dental teams need to be aware of and be able to respond to patients' concerns so that they both accept and value radiographs as a meaningful and necessary diagnostic tool.

Payors often limit the number or type of radiographs paid for each benefit year. Refunds are required if an audit reveals radiographs were taken unnecessarily, if the radiographs do not meet the recognized quality standard, or if the dentist never specifically ordered or read them (as noted in the dental record).

The American Dental Association (ADA), in cooperation with the Food and Drug Administration (FDA), established guidelines for the exposure to dental radiographs in 1987 (with subsequent revisions in 2004) and made recommendations subject to the dentist's clinical judgment on best practice regarding the approach of diagnostic imaging on an individual patient basis. The dentist must use professional judgment, a thorough clinical evaluation, consider multiple risk factors, and review the patient's health history to determine the best use of diagnostic imaging for each patient. Treatment recommendations, including radiographs, should not be dependant on frequency limitations of insurance plans, but rather based on medical necessity. The doctor should prescribe radiographs based on need, not reimbursement. Never write "Pt. was not due for radiographs" in the chart notes, as it implies treatment based on frequency, not medical neccessity.

Because every precaution should be taken to minimize radiation exposure, protective thyroid collars and aprons should be used whenever possible. This practice is strongly recommended for children, women of childbearing age, and pregnant women.

Dental practitioners use radiographic images for a variety of purposes. Radiographs can help identify caries in a tooth or provide the location of an impacted tooth that needs to be extracted. Depending on the purpose of the radiograph, the dental practitioner may choose to utilize one of the two major categories of dental radiographs: intraoral or extraoral.

An intraoral radiograph utilizes a film or sensor positioned inside the mouth during image capture. On the contrary, with extraoral images, the film or sensor is positioned outside of the mouth during image capture.

Intraoral Radiographs

Intraoral radiographs are the most common type of dental radiographic image because they provide significant detail. Among other things, these radiographic images allow the dentist to identify caries, check the health of the tooth root(s) and the bone surrounding the tooth/teeth, determine the status of developing teeth, and monitor the general health of the teeth and other hard tissue structures.

The advent of tomosynthesis as a diagnostic tool in dentistry will further add to the clinician's armamentarium. Stationary Intraoral Tomosynthesis (sIOT) uses multiple x-ray focal sources in slightly different angulations in a single exposure, with an intraoral sensor capable of detecting each source and creating an image "stack". These multiple images are then combined with a computer algorithm to create a 3 dimensional image. This image allows for a clinician to scroll through layers of the tooth looking for pathology, including caries, and anatomical features such as multiple canals. The radiograph unit and sensor are similar to traditional radiograph heads and digital sensors while yielding significantly more information than a two dimensional image.

Extraoral Radiographs

While extraoral radiographs display the teeth, their function and focus is often more general in nature than that of intraoral radiographs. In the past, traditional extraoral radiographs did not provide the same level of detail as intraoral radiographs, so they were rarely used to detect cavities or identify problems with individual teeth. Instead, extraoral radiographs were used to screen for impacted teeth or infections, to monitor growth and development of the jaws in relation to the teeth, and to identify potential relational issues between the teeth and jaws and the temporomandibular joint. However, developing extraoral technology is changing this usage, making these images similar in resolution to intraoral images. In addition, the integration of CBCT into every day dental practice is now a valuable tool for diagnosis and treatment planning, including evaluating maxillofacial anatomy and planning implant placement.

Clinical situations for which radiographs may be indicated include, but are not limited to:

Positive Historical Findings

1. Previous periodontal or endodontic treatment

2. History of pain or trauma

3. Familial history of dental anomalies

4. Postoperative evaluation of healing

5. Remineralization monitoring

6. Presence of implants, previous implant related pathosis, or evaluation for implant placement

Positive Clinical Signs/ Symptoms:

1. Clinical evidence of periodontal disease

2. Large or deep restorations

3. Deep carious lesions

4. Malposed or clinically impacted teeth

5. Swelling

6. Evidence of dental/facial trauma

7. Mobility of teeth

8. Sinus tract ("fistula")

9. Clinically suspected sinus pathosis

10. Growth abnormalities

11. Oral involvement in known or suspected systemic disease

12. Positive neurologic findings in the head and neck

13. Evidence of foreign objects

14. Pain and/or dysfunction of the temporomandibular joint

15. Facial asymmetry

16. Abutment teeth for fixed or removable partial prosthesis

17. Unexplained bleeding

18. Unexplained sensitivity of teeth

19. Unusual eruption, spacing, or migration of teeth

20. Unusual tooth morphology, calcification, or color

21. Unexplained absence of teeth

22. Clinical tooth erosion

23. Peri-implantitis

**Factors increasing risk for caries may be assessed using the ADA Caries Risk Assessment forms (zero–six years of age and over six years of age).* Access these using the URL and password on the inside front cover.

The standard of care dictates that radiographs should be taken only when necessary. Therefore, it is inappropriate to routinely take radiographs simply because payors reimburse them at certain time intervals. The following should be considered when developing radiograph protocols for your practice:

1. Radiographs should only be ordered by a dentist (or hygienist if state permits evaluations, diagnosis, and/or treatment plans by a hygienist). Routine practice protocols should never be determined solely based on an established interval of time between radiographs (e.g., four BW once per year for all adults). Contributing factors as previously listed, as well as caries risk assessment may increase or decrease

the frequency of diagnostic radiographs. For supervision levels of permitted services by state, visit https://www.adha.org/resources-docs/7511_Permitted_Services_Supervision_Levels_by_State.pdf

As always, verify information with your State Dental Board to ensure you are in compliance.

2. Rather than having set office protocols where certain radiographs are always taken, best practice is for radiographs to be ordered after performing a preliminary examination of the patient and assessing the need. The preliminary examination and decision to expose the patient to radiation should be determined and ordered in writing by a licensed dental professional. Various conditions and situations (as outlined in the ADA/FDA guidelines) when observed in a patient, may justify the increased frequency of taking radiographs.

3. Radiographs should only be ordered when they are deemed necessary for the proper diagnosis and treatment of a potentially pathologic condition. Justification for taking a radiograph must be recorded in the patient's clinical record. The positive signs and symptoms (and caries risk factors) listed above may be used to establish the necessity and frequency for radiographs.

4. Radiographs should only be ordered after the patient has been informed of the benefits and risks of radiograph exposure and patient consent has been received and noted in the clinical record.

5. Radiographs should be taken in a manner that keeps exposure to a minimum. Proper team training will help ensure that the radiographic image is of diagnostic quality and is obtained with the least number of retakes.

6. Radiographs should be reviewed thoroughly and observations noted in the clinical record. When radiographs are taken, an entry indicating that they were reviewed/interpreted must also be noted in the clinical record. The chart entry must include the radiographic findings, even when they are negative. If radiographs are not reviewed, an insurance auditor may determine that reimbursement is not warranted since CDT codes for radiographs typically include interpretation and have a higher reimbursement. If the clinical record does not include a notation that the radiographs were reviewed and interpreted from a legal standpoint, it did not happen.

7. Radiographs should be properly maintained and readily available for review with minimal effort or delay.

8. Radiographs should be of diagnostic quality (no overlapping contacts, cone cutting, or cut off apices). Proper diagnosis cannot occur without quality radiographs. In addition, submitting non-diagnostic radiographs to payors may flag a practice for an audit, as these radiographs are not reimbursable.

Patient Scenario:

Mrs. Madisen Ireland, a new adult patient arrives in the office. A detailed dental and medical history is completed by the patient using the standard practice questionnaire, followed by a patient interview to clarify any points of concern. Additional details per patient history:

- Patient is a 53-year-old, moderately obese, white female.

- She reveals that she does not floss and brushes only once per day.

- She has not been to the dentist for treatment of any kind for 8 years. Her last visit was to have an infected wisdom tooth extracted.

- Patient reveals her husband complains that she has bad breath constantly.

- Her medical history indicates that she is being treated for elevated cholesterol and high blood pressure.

- She had a tonsillectomy in 1969 and an appendectomy in 1972.

- She admits to having smoked a pack of cigarettes a day until 11 years ago, but quit in 2001 because "her doctor scared her into quitting."

The patient's dental history indicates a high risk of dental disease. A brief examination by the dentist reveals generalized red swollen gingiva, visible active decay present in four teeth, a noticeable periodontal odor, and a PSR screening of threes. The findings of a caries risk assessment are high risk. The dentist determines a high probability of moderate to severe periodontitis.

Using the ADA/FDA guidelines found at the end of this chapter on Page 26, this patient would be classified across the top column as Adult, Dentate or Partially Edentulous. The patient would also be classified down the left column as a New Patient being evaluated for oral diseases. Therefore, the protocol in the box that intersects with the column titled Adult Dentate or Partially Edentulous and New Patient being evaluated for oral diseases suggests that (an) "Individualized radiographic exam (be completed) consisting of posterior bitewings with panoramic exam or posterior bitewings and selected periapical images." It also states, "A full mouth intraoral radiographic exam is preferred when the patient has clinical evidence of generalized oral disease or a history of extensive dental treatment."

A full mouth intraoral radiographic series should be the standard of care for this patient according to the ADA/ FDA radiographic guidelines because there is evidence of generalized dental disease.

The explanation written in the patient's clinical notes for taking the full mouth series might be: "Significant evidence of generalized dental disease. Initial screening oral examination revealed visible areas of decay, periodontal pocketing, bleeding on probing, and other factors that suggest more information is necessary. A full series of radiographs is necessary in order to provide a complete and thorough diagnosis of the location, severity, and types of disease present."

All dental practices should be familiar with the ADA/FDA radiographic guidelines and utilize them as a foundation for establishing appropriate radiographs based on each patient's specific situation. Note that these recommendations are subject to clinical judgment and may not apply to every patient. Whenever possible, every attempt should be made to reduce/minimize a patient's exposure to dental radiographs. Team training should be conducted on a regular basis to help eliminate retakes and to ensure a high diagnostic quality of radiographs. This is a goal that should be shared and communicated by every dental practice and one that will be appreciated by all patients.

Notes

Type of Encounter	Patient Age and Dental Developmental Stage				
	Child with Primary Dentition (prior to eruption of first permanent tooth)	**Child with Transitional Dentition (after eruption of first permanent tooth)**	**Adolescent with Permanent Dentition (prior to eruption of third molars)**	**Adult, Dentate or Partially Edentulous**	**Adult, Edentulous**
New Patient* being evaluated for oral diseases	Individualized radiographic exam consisting of selected periapical/occlusal views and/or posterior bitewings if proximal surfaces cannot be visualized or probed. Patients without evidence of disease and with open proximal contacts may not require a radiographic exam at this time.	Individualized radiographic exam consisting of posterior bitewings with panoramic exam or posterior bitewings and selected periapical images.	Individualized radiographic exam consisting of posterior bitewings with panoramic exam or posterior bitewings and selected periapical images. A full mouth intraoral radiographic exam is preferred when the patient has clinical evidence of generalized oral disease or a history of extensive dental treatment.		Individualized radiographic exam, based on clinical signs and symptoms.
Recare Patient* with clinical caries or at increased risk for caries**	Posterior bitewing exam at 6-12 month intervals if proximal surfaces cannot be examined visually or with a probe.			Posterior bitewing exam at 6-18 month intervals.	Not applicable.
Recare Patient* with no clinical caries and not at increased risk for caries**	Posterior bitewing exam at 12-24 month intervals if proximal surfaces cannot be examined visually or with a probe.		Posterior bitewing exam at 18-36 month intervals.	Posterior bitewing exam at 24-36 month intervals.	Not applicable.
Recare Patient* with periodontal disease	Clinical judgment as to the need for and type of radiographic images for the evaluation of periodontal disease. Imaging may consist of, but is not limited to, selected bitewing and/or periapical images of areas where periodontal disease (other than nonspecific gingivitis) can be demonstrated clinically.				Not applicable.
Patient (New and Recare) for monitoring of dentofacial growth and development, and/or assessment of dental/skeletal relationships	Clinical judgment as to need for and type of radiographic images for evaluation and/or monitoring of dentofacial growth and development or assessment of dental and skeletal relationships.		Clinical judgment as to need for and type of radiographic images for evaluation and/or monitoring of dentofacial growth and development, or assessment of dental and skeletal relationships. Panoramic or periapical exam to assess developing third molars.	Usually not indicated for monitoring of growth and development. Clinical judgment as to the need for and type of radiographic image for evaluation of dental and skeletal relationships.	
Patient with other circumstances including, but not limited to, proposed or existing implants, other dental and craniofacial pathoses, restorative/endodontic needs, treated periodontal disease and caries remineralization	Clinical judgment as to need for and type of radiographic images for evaluation and/or monitoring of these conditions.				

Notes

Record retention guidelines vary widely, depending on your state of residence, as well as your unique tax situation.

Patient Records and Records Retention

Record retention guidelines vary widely, depending on your state of residence, as well as your unique tax situation. Before destroying or discarding patient records and/or business records, it is important to review your state laws and consult with your accountant regarding financial record retention, as well as to check with your state dental board regarding rules for patient record retention. To follow are some general guidelines. Any patient information committed to paper must be shredded before discarding.

Patient Records

Requirements for the length of time required for retaining patient records varies widely by state. Most states require doctors to retain records for at least six years from the date of the patient's last appointment. However, be aware that some states require doctors to retain patient records for a longer period of time (seven to ten years). Records for minors are usually retained for at least six years beyond reaching the age of 18. Doctors should verify their state's dental regulations and if the state has no patient records retention directive, then they should reach out to their malpractice carrier for direction. Additionally, once the mandated time frame expires, it is up to the provider to decide how long to retain patient records. Federal programs, such as Medicare, also have record retention policies that must be followed.

Patient requests for records and/or radiographs should be in writing with specific instructions on where to send the records. Some states allow a copying fee (usually reasonable costs, not exceeding actual costs, incurred by the dental office for providing these copies) to be charged to the patient. Keep in mind, however, that the Health Insurance Portability and Accountability Act (HIPAA) Privacy Rule does not allow Covered Entities to charge a fee for retrieving records. The amount doctors are allowed to charge for copying records also varies widely from state to state and is often updated to reflect inflation. You should also be aware of your state regulations regarding the time frame for providing the requested information.

Doctors may not withhold patient records due to an outstanding balance on a patient's account as this is a violation of the HIPAA Privacy Rule. Before withholding patient records, it is best to check with your state licensing board to ensure you are in compliance with state law and not at risk of losing your license. In addition, withholding records due to an outstanding balance on a patient's account violates the ADA's Code of Ethics, found at www.ada.org/en/about-the-ada/principles-of-ethics-code-of-professional-conduct

Electronic Records

In today's electronic age, an increasing number of dental practices are "paperless," thus making it easier to maintain records for longer periods of time. It is imperative that electronic records are backed up regularly and a copy is kept off-site so that they are easily retrieved, if necessary.

With each state or territory having their own unique laws, consult with your accountant, state dental association, state board, and malpractice carrier regarding proper record retention for your individual state. ıl

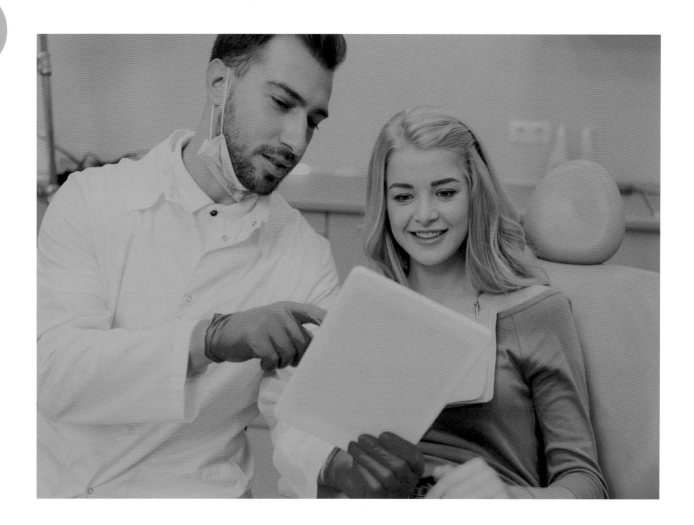

Notes

The Health Insurance Portability and Accountability Act of 1996, is a federal law that sets forth national standards to protect patient health information from being disclosed without the patient's consent or knowledge.

CHAPTER SEVEN

HIPAA and Cyber Security

The Office of Civil Rights within the Department of Human Services (HHS) is the governing body for the Health Insurance Portability and Accountability Act, commonly called HIPAA.

The Health Insurance Portability and Accountability Act of 1996, is a federal law that sets forth national standards to protect patient health information from being disclosed without the patient's consent or knowledge. HIPAA has two main components; the HIPAA Privacy Rule and the HIPAA Security Rule.

According to HHS.gov, "The HIPAA Privacy Rule establishes national standards to protect individuals' medical records and other individually identifiable health information (collectively defined as "protected health information") and applies to health plans, health care clearinghouses, and those health care providers that conduct certain health care transactions electronically. The Rule requires appropriate safeguards to protect the privacy of protected health information and sets limits and conditions on the uses and disclosures that may be made of such information without an individual's authorization. The Rule also gives individuals rights over their protected health information, including rights to examine and obtain a copy of their health records, to direct a covered entity to transmit to a third party an electronic copy of their protected health information in an electronic health record, and to request corrections."

"The HIPAA Security Rule establishes national standards to protect individuals' electronic personal health information that is created, received, used, or maintained by a covered entity. The Security Rule requires appropriate administrative, physical and technical safeguards to ensure the confidentiality, integrity, and security of electronic protected health information."

With the recent update to the 21st Century Cures 2.0 Act, clear and precise patient records are more important than ever. Patients will soon be able to see their patient records with the ability to access online at any given time. The rule is designed to give access to patients and other associated healthcare providers to secure electronic health information (EHO), aka patient records. These changes are ever-evolving. Refer to www.practicebooster.com/documentation for updates throughout the year (password located on inside front cover).

Key Terms to Remember

- Covered Entity (CE) − includes:

  − A health plan

  − A health care clearinghouses

  − A health care provider who transmits any health information in electronic form

- NPP − Notice of Privacy Practices

- Business Associate (BA) − anyone a covered entity does business with

- Breach − generally defined as an impermissible use or disclosure

A breach can occur in various ways. It is important to remember that all patient information is confidential and should remain that way. According to HIPAA regulations, the person committing the breach will be responsible for and held accountable for any infractions that may occur. This could result in huge fines and even jail time, depending on the severity of the breach.

Rise of Privacy Complaints and Cyber Security Issues

Privacy complaints and cyber security issues have risen significantly since the passage of HIPAA. As of June 2021, the OCR has received over 267,736 complaints since the agency began enforcing the Privacy Rule in April 2003.

These statistics reveal that patients are exercising their legal rights more often by filing privacy complaints with the OCR. The increasing rate of complaints based upon oversights, mishaps, carelessness, or negligence, shows that there is nothing administratively simple about this Act, nor is compliance something to take lightly.

If a patient has a privacy complaint, invite the patient to meet with your Privacy Officer to discuss the situation and complete your privacy complaint form (not to be filed with the patient record). Ideally, the matter can be resolved internally, and the patient will not file a complaint with the Office of Civil Rights (OCR). Like all consumers, patients want their complaints heard and validated; they want an apology and an earnest attempt to resolve the situation.

Complaints involving BAs can be even more complicated. For example, one patient discovered their before-and-after treatment radiographs (not actual patient photographs) had been published on the practice's new website without their permission. The web design company's test site accidentally went live. Anyone surfing the Internet could view the patient's protected information. The patient filed a privacy complaint with OCR.

According to a U.S. Government Interagency technical guidance document, since 2016 over 4,000 ransomware attacks have happened daily in the U.S. Protecting your practice from cyber security threats is more important than ever. The newest federal law to address this ever-growing issue is the HIPAA Safe Harbor Rule. Signed into law in January 2021, the HIPAA Safe Harbor Rule amended the HITECH Act requiring HHS to incentivize cybersecurity best practices for CEs and BAs for fulfilling their HIPAA obligations. This means that the HHS will consider whether a CE or BA has adequately demonstrated that recognized security practices have been in place for at least 12 months and will reduce the potential penalties which might have otherwise been implemented as a result of potential HIPAA Security Rule violations. Under this Bill, recognized security practices are defined as "standards, guidelines, best practices, methodologies, procedures, and processes developed under section 2(c)(15) of the National Institute of Standards and Technology Act, the approaches promulgated under section 405(d) of the Cybersecurity Act of 2015 (CSA), and other programs and processes that address cybersecurity and that are developed, recognized, or promulgated through regulations under other statutory authorities."

In addition, if a breach of unsecured PHI occurred and it affected fewer than 500 individuals, you must notify HHS of the breach within 60 days of the end of the calendar year in which the breach was discovered. For a breach affecting more than 500 individuals, you must notify HHS without unreasonable delay and in no case later than 60 days following a breach. Unsecure information is considered any patient data that has not been made unreadable or indecipherable to unauthorized individuals through a specified technology or methodology such as encryption.

For more information on HIPAA requirements and Cyber Security, please refer to Practice Booster's, *Dental Administration With Confidence.*

Notes

Since we never know when or if the documentation will need to be recalled, it is important to paint a detailed picture of what took place.

Documenting Clinical Treatment and Procedures

Guidelines

Documenting services creates a visual road map of what has taken place on any given day. It is important to record every procedure with detail. Since we never know when or if the documentation will need to be recalled, it is important to paint a detailed picture of what took place.

This section will review and give examples of documentation for various services and provide an example of S.O.A.P. notes for each one. For the actual CDT codes, you will need to refer to Practice Booster's *Dental Coding With Confidence.*

Detailed documentation of all services serves two purposes, first; in the event of a malpractice suit, our documentation becomes evidence in a court of law or dental board. Second, it serves as a baseline for all future appointments. You can get a much broader understanding of a patient when your documentation is thorough.

When reporting any service, it is important to carefully review a patient's medical and dental history since their last visit. Since patients do not always understand the link between oral and systemic health, it is important to ask them open-ended questions and avoid questions they can answer with a simple "yes" or "no". Questions like: "When was the last time you were in the emergency room?" or "When was the last time your doctor changed your medication?" are open-ended questions and will get you more detailed answers. Oftentimes the answers from these questions, will lead you to more in-depth questions where you will get a better understanding of their overall medical/dental history. Important things to review may include:

- Medications
- Past or recent illnesses
- Diabetes
- Cancers throughout the body
- Blood Pressure
- Cardiovascular issues
- Allergies
- Immune deficiency
- Sinus issues
- Anything on their medical history that needs further investigation
- If patient has a history of smoking, drug use or alcohol abuse
- Changes in diet

Not only is it imperative to report findings, but to bring it to the dentist's attention prior to proceeding with treatment should one of these circumstances create a need for treatment to be delayed.

At each visit, the medical history should be **reviewed, signed and dated** as documentation that it was reviewed. If a patient fails to disclose a condition or medication they may have taken, their signature will serve as a record of the conditions they have disclosed.

S.O.A.P. Notes

To recap, SOAP stands for:

- **Subjective** — Chief complaint by the patient and observation of condition

- **Objective** — Data collected that you see, hear and what the patient feels, taste, smells

- **Assessment** — Diagnosis is made

- **Plan** — create a plan or options available to the patient

S.O.A.P. NOTE BASIC TEMPLATE

Basic Template:

Disclaimer: This template serves solely as a guide and may not include all information applicable to every procedural charting. This template does not serve as legal advice. If you are in need of legal counsel, be sure to contact a licensed healthcare attorney.

Use the relevant sections of this template and remove the rest. This template is a guide and may not include all information applicable to every procedural charting. Add appropriate information as needed. As always, be as thorough as possible. Including more information is always better than leaving things out.

Date: _____ Time: _____ Dr: _____

SUBJECTIVE FINDINGS ─────────────────────────────────── **S**

Reason For Visit/Chief Complaint: **Dental History:**

Medical History: **Social History:**

OBJECTIVE FINDINGS ─────────────────────────────────── **O**

Vitals: Clinical Exam

BP: _____   **Radiographs:**

Pulse: _____   **Extraoral Exam:**

Temp: _____   **Intraoral Exam:**

Blood Glucose Level: _____

ASSESSMENT ─────────────────────────────────── **A**

Periodontal Condition: **Hard tissue condition:**

PLAN ─────────────────────────────────── **P**

Treatment rendered today: **Next visit:**

Rx: Assistant:

     Treating Dentist:

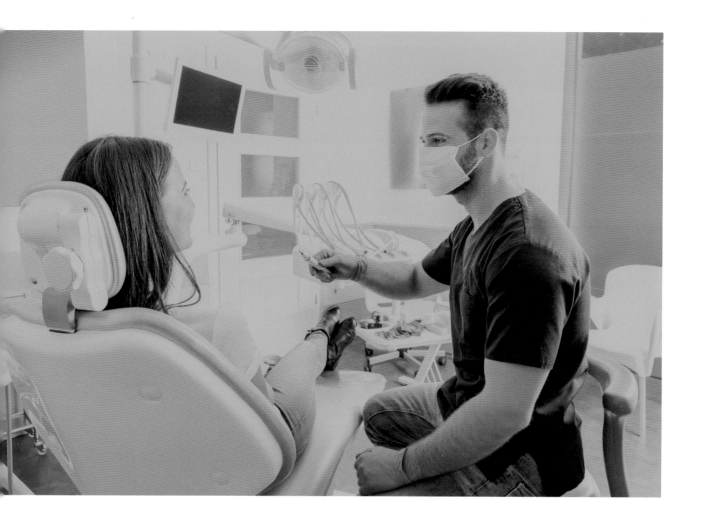

Charting Diagnostic Procedures

Be thorough in reporting each diagnostic service performed. Record all visual findings as even the slightest finding could be a baseline for evaluations down the road. Records should include:

- Date

- Vital signs

- Existing restorations — if not noted

- New cavities

- Fractures

- Mobile teeth

- Evidence of weakening of existing restorations; open margins, cracked fillings, leakage around restorations, erosion, etc.

- Any discomfort or complications

- Bone or gingival recession

- Evidence of bruxism, or TMJ disorders

- Offset of bite

- Visual exam of lips, oral mucosa, and tongue

- Any and all radiographs that were taken and intra-oral pictures

- Next visit recommendations

Comprehensive Oral Evaluation / **Date:** 4/23/2023 **Time:** 9:30 AM **Dr:** M. Nice

SUBJECTIVE FINDINGS

Reason For Visit/Chief Complaint:

The patient, a 23 y.o. male, presented to Dr. Nice for initial evaluation, accompanied by his girlfriend. Pt stated he was happy with his smile but had "a little soreness on (his) gums on the upper right side" which has presented intermittently for six months. Pt stated he was "scared of what (we) may find." Pt also asked about tooth whitening.

Medical History:

Medical history intake form was reviewed. Pt has no significant medical conditions.

No current medications are being taken.

NKDA

Dental History:

Pt has not seen a dentist in three years. He stated he did not have a good experience at his last dental office. He stated it "hurt when (he) had (his) teeth cleaned."

Social History:

Pt smokes 1 pack of cigarettes weekly.

Social alcohol use averaging 3-4 beers per week, usually on the weekends only.

No recreational drug use was reported.

OBJECTIVE FINDINGS

Vitals:
BP: 120/80
Pulse: 80
Temp: 98

Clinical Exam

Radiographs:

After a cursory exam, Dr. Nice requested a comprehensive series of radiographs (FMX) including 14 PAs and 4 BWs. Radiographs were necessary for a baseline assessment and to develop an accurate treatment plan.

Radiographs were then reviewed by Dr. Nice and suspected areas of decay and bone loss were noted.

Extraoral Exam:

Oral cancer screening (OCS) was performed.
No facial swelling or asymmetry was noted.

No tenderness on palpation on the face, neck, or jaw joints.

No pain or crepitus was noted with jaw movements in TMJ evaluation.

Intraoral Exam:

Oral cancer screening (OCS) was performed including the use of Velscope with no areas of concern.

A comprehensive oral evaluation was completed by Dr. Nice, including charting existing restorations, missing teeth, and areas of concern.

Complete periodontal charting and probing were also completed.

Intraoral (IO) photos were taken to support clinical observations. The patient was shown the photos in an effort to educate them and enroll them in care. Pt acknowledged the areas of concern.

ASSESSMENT   A

Periodontal Condition:

Overall gingival tissue health appeared poor.

Inflammation was noted around teeth #2-#5 with bleeding on probing.

Patient has moderate plaque, light calculus, but heavy staining from smoking.

Pocket depths are ≤ 3mm with no bone loss.

Localized, moderate gingivitis in the upper right posterior quadrant.

Hard tissue condition:

Caries Risk Assessment: Moderate (Questionnaire on file)

Small areas of interproximal decay are present in the UR quadrant as detected on radiographs.

PLAN   P

Treatment rendered today:

Comprehensive oral evaluation
FMX
OCS
Velscope
Caries Risk Assessment
IO photos
No prescriptions given

Future treatment required includes:

D1110 prophylaxis — adult
D1206 Fl varnish
D2392 MO tooth #3
D2392 DO tooth #4

Rx:

No prescriptions given.

Next visit:

Prophy with focus on the UR quadrant
Fl varnish

Assistant: E. Sential
Treating Dentist: M. Nice

Notes

_____

_____

_____

_____

_____

_____

_____

_____

_____

_____

_____

_____

Charting Hygiene Procedures

The examples given in **Diagnostic Services** will also be recorded each time a patient presents for re-care in order to establish any abnormalities or changes that have occurred since their last visit. In addition, the following things should be recorded as well:

- Consent form signed

- Medical history reviewed signed and dated

- Risk of carious diseases

- Periodontal probing depths (six recordings per tooth)

- Bleeding, specify area(s)

- Type of fluoride given (when applicable)

- Any oral recommendations/medications given

- Excessive plaque or calculus present

- Oral health home care instructions given

- Sealant recommendations (where applicable) and material used

- Any new radiographs or intra-oral pictures taken

- Any study models taken (where applicable)

- Any complications that occurred or the fact that none occurred

- Next visit recommendations

Recare Appointment / **Date:** 4/23/2023 **Time:** 9:00 AM **Dr:** A. Sample

SUBJECTIVE FINDINGS S

Reason For Visit/Chief Complaint:

Pt., a 42 y.o. male, presents for a routine preventive visit, accompanied by his wife. Pt complains of sensitivity in his UR quadrant.

Medical History: Medical Hx was reviewed with no changes since the last visit.

Dental History: Pt. was last seen for routine dental prophylaxis in our office on 10/20/2022.

OBJECTIVE FINDINGS O

Vitals:

BP: 120/80   Pulse: 80   Temp: 98

Clinical Exam

Radiographs:After a cursory exam, Dr. Sample ordered four BWs to check for interproximal decay and one PA of tooth #3 to look for periapical pathology.

Radiographs were then reviewed by Dr. Sample.

Extraoral Exam: Oral cancer screening was performed.

No facial swelling or asymmetry was noted. No tenderness on palpation on the face, neck, or jaw joints.

No pain or crepitus was noted with jaw movements in TMJ evaluation.

Intraoral Exam: Oral cancer screening (OCS) was performed including the use of Velscope with no areas of concern.

Dr. Sample performed a periodic oral evaluation.

ASSESSMENT A

Periodontal Condition:

Overall gingival tissue appeared healthy.

Patient has moderate plaque and light calculus.

Pocket depths are ≤ 3mm.

Endodontic Condition:

Decay noted on the mesial of tooth #3 extending into the dentin.

PLAN P

Prophylaxis is needed to remove plaque, calculus, and stains from tooth structures with the intent to control local irritational factors.

Fluoride (Fl) varnish was recommended due to moderate caries risk assessment to assist in preventing caries.

Treatment rendered today:

Prophy including supragingival hand scaling and polishing with rubber cup.

4 BW
1 PA- #3
Periodic oral evaluation
OCS
Velscope
Fl varnish

Oral hygiene instruction was given including brushing instruction and a flossing demonstration.

Reviewed treatment needed at next visit (MO #3).

Rx:

No prescriptions given.

Next visit:

MO composite resin on tooth #3.

Next Hyg visit: 6 mo

Hyg: D. Bride
Assistant: R. Hand
Treating Dentist: A. Sample

Charting Periodontal Therapy

Periodontal therapy is a non-surgical treatment for gum disease that usually includes scaling and root planing (SRP) to remove subgingival tartar, calculus, and infected dentin. The clinical note must be thorough and complete to support a SRP claim. Records should include the following:

- Date of procedure
- Medical history was reviewed, signed and dated
- Medical condition that may be a contributing factor to condition
- Patient's vital signs (pre and post op)
- Consent form signed
- Any issues the patient may be experiencing
- Full mouth radiographs to support claim
- Probing depths (six points per tooth)
- Diagnosis of periodontitis (i.e., generalized, chronic, moderate)
- Description of periodontitis (i.e., location of bleeding points, purulent discharge, increase in pocket depth, loss of attachment, recession, mobility, etc.)
- Note that both scaling and root planing were both performed in certain areas
- Procedure performed
- Bleeding, specify area
- Clinical attachment loss (See note below)
- Any medications or pre-medications taken
- Type(s) and amount of anesthetic used
- Post care instructions given
- Any recommendations given
- Post medications given (where applicable)
- Any new radiographs or intra-oral pictures taken

- Any complications that occurred or the fact that none occurred
- Next visit recommendations

Clinical Attachment Loss (CAL)

Clinical attachment loss occurs as a result of recession and bone loss due to periodontal disease. The amount of CAL, if any, must be clearly documented in the patient's chart in order to support the need for treatment. CAL can be calculated by comparing the position of the gingival margin to the cementoenamel junction (CEJ), which is the point where the enamel surface meets the cementum surface of the root.

1. The gingival margin may be at the cementoenamel junction (CEJ). In that case, the pocket depth equals the CAL.

2. The gingival margin may be coronal to (covering) the CEJ. In that case, the distance between the gingival margin and the CEJ must be subtracted from the pocket depth to determine the CAL.

3. The gingival margin may be apical to (not covering) the CEJ (i.e., the CEJ is visible). In that case the distance from the CEJ to the gingival margin must be added to the pocket depth to determine the CAL.

PERIODONTAL THERAPY S.O.A.P. NOTE EXAMPLE

SRP / **Date:** 4/23/2023 **Time:** 9:30 AM **Dr:** C. Gracey

SUBJECTIVE FINDINGS
S

Reason For Visit/Chief Complaint:

The patient, a 40 y.o. male, presents for periodontal scaling and root planing.

Medical History: Reviewed medical history. No change since last visit.

Social History: Pt has smoked 1 pack/day since 2002.

Dental History: Right side scaled and root planed on 4/10/2023.

Left side scaled and root planed today.

OBJECTIVE FINDINGS
O

Vitals:

BP: 120/80   Pulse: 80   Temp: 98

Clinical Exam

Radiographs:

Relevant radiographs taken 3/15/2023. No new radiographs required today.

Intraoral Exam:

Generalized 2-5mm pockets.

CAL noted on perio charting with bleeding on probing.

Generalized moderate bone loss and subgingival calculus noted on radiographs.

Class I mobility on teeth #14, #18, and #19.

ASSESSMENT
A

Periodontal Condition:

AAP stage 2, grade B, active moderate periodontitis

PLAN
P

Nonsurgical SRP quadrants II and III

Treatment rendered today:

The procedure was explained. Alternatives and risks were discussed. Pt. had no questions and consented to treatment.

Topical anesthetic placed. 3 carpules of Numbocaine 4% 1:100,000 with epi injected using a 30- gauge short needle into maxillary buccal vestibule left side.

2 carpules of Numbocaine 4% 1:100,000 with epi injected using a 27- gauge long needle IAN.

Aspiration was negative.

The patient tolerated the injections and had no adverse reactions. Anesthesia was achieved.

Calculus was removed from supragingival and subgingival surfaces of UL and LL quadrants using an ultrasonic scaler followed by hand instruments. Heavy bleeding around upper and lower posterior teeth. Significant nicotine staining around lower anteriors.

Pt tolerated treatment well.

OHI was given, including instructions on chlorhexidine rinse,

brushing, and flossing. Pt was informed of the correlation between smoking and periodontal issues/oral cancer.

Rx:

Prescriptions were given to help manage oral bacteria.

Chlorhexidine mouth rinse, 1 bottle; rinse with 30 ml once/day.

Next visit:

Perio maintenance in 90 days

Hyg: D. Bride
Treating Dentist: C. Gracey

8

Charting Restorative Procedures

When a patient presents for restorative treatment, vital signs should be taken and compared to baseline data taken at previous appointments. Any abnormalities should be directed to the doctor before the procedure gets underway.

Your notes should include:

- Date of procedure

- Medical history was reviewed, signed and dated

- Patient's vital signs (pre and post op)

- Consent form signed

- Any issues the patient may be experiencing in that area

- Procedure performed

- Any medications taken

- Type and amount of anesthetic used

- Material used; bases, liners, bond, filling material

- Rubber dam use and clamp size (when applicable)

- Any new radiographs or intra-oral pictures taken

- Post care instructions given

- Post medications given (where applicable)

- Any complications that occurred or the fact that none occurred

- Next visit recommendations

Nitrous Oxide

Documentation of the use of nitrous oxide must be made in chart notes much like any other medication given to the patient. All information should be noted completely and accurately. In addition to your restorative notes, these things should be recorded:

- Consent form for nitrous oxide signed and dated

- Maximum level of nitrous oxide/oxygen used in terms of percentages or each gas used and total volume used

- Duration of administration

- Length of oxygenation

- Patient's report of feeling "normal" prior to dismissal

- Any complication occurred or the fact that none occurred

Posterior Composite Fillings / **Date:** 4/23/2023 **Time:** 2:30 PM **Dr:** A. Smiles

SUBJECTIVE FINDINGS — S

Reason For Visit/Chief Complaint:

The patient, a 16 y.o. male, presents for composite restorations on teeth #13, #14, #19, and #20, accompanied by his mother. Pt. states he is "kind of scared" and wants "gas".

Medical History: Medical Hx was reviewed with no changes since the last visit.

Dental History: Patient had a comprehensive exam on 02/03/2023 which showed signs of interproximal decay in posterior on both sides.

OBJECTIVE FINDINGS — O

Vitals:

BP: 110/70   Pulse: 60   Temp: 98

Clinical Exam

Radiographs:

Relevant radiographs taken 02/03/2023.
No new radiographs necessary.

ASSESSMENT — A

N2O required to help mitigate patient anxiety.

Composite resin restorations required to replace decayed tooth structure and stop caries progression.

PLAN — P

Composite resin restorations on DO #13, MO #14, MO #19, DO #20

Treatment rendered today:

The procedure was explained. Alternatives and risks were discussed. Pt. had no questions and consented to treatment. Consent form was signed.

N2O-given at 40%. Started at 2:45 PM. Stopped at 3:22 PM.

Topical anesthetic placed. 1 carpule of Numbocaine 4% 1:100,000 with epi injected using a 30- gauge short needle into buccal vestibule above tooth #14.

1 carpules of Numbocaine 4% 1:100,000 with epi injected using a 27- gauge long needle IAN. Aspiration was negative for both injections.

The patient tolerated the injections and had no adverse reactions. Anesthesia was achieved.

Upper left quadrant isolated using a rubber dam. Decay was removed. Placed matrix band and wedge. Teeth prepared using SelfEtching Bond 2 and light cured. FlowBul flowable resin placed on prep floor and light cured. PackIT composite resin placed in increments and light cured to restore form and function.

Lower left quadrant isolated using rubber dam. Decay was removed. Placed matrix band and wedge. Teeth prepared using SelfEtching Bond 2 and light cured. FlowBul flowable resin placed on prep floor and light cured. PackIT composite resin placed in increments and light cured to restore form and function.

Decay was deep on tooth #19. Informed the patient of the possibility of cold sensitivity, but if pain occurs to contact our office. Prognosis is good.

Occlusion adjusted and contacts checked.

100% O2 given for 5 minutes. Pt's mental, physical, and emotional condition returned to normal prior to dismissal.

Verbal post op instructions reviewed with pt and his mom. Pt tolerated treatment well.

Rx: No prescriptions given.

Next visit: Restorations on right side.

Assistant: A. Helper
Treating Dentist: A. Smiles

Root canal therapy is done when bacteria infiltrate the tooth or trauma has occurred within the tooth causing it to "die". The inflamed pulp of the tooth is removed, the canal cleaned, sterilized, filled, and sealed. Important to note are the size files and final size of the canal before filling. Include the following:

- Date of procedure

- Medical history was reviewed, signed and dated

- Patient's vital signs (pre and post op)

- Consent form signed

- Any issues the patient may be experiencing in that area

- Procedure performed

- Any medications taken

- Type and amount of anesthetic used

- Material used; irrigations solutions, type of obturate used, sealers

- Rubber dam use and clamp size (when applicable)

- Any new radiographs or intra-oral pictures taken

- Post care instructions given

- Post medications given (where applicable)

- Any complications that occurred or the fact that none occurred

- Next visit recommendations

ENDODONTICS S.O.A.P NOTE EXAMPLE

Premolar RCT / **Date:** 4/23/2023 **Time:** 11:00 AM **Dr:** N. Doh

SUBJECTIVE FINDINGS ──────────────────────────── S

Reason For Visit/Chief Complaint:

The patient, a 50 y.o. female, presents for endodontic therapy on tooth #5. Pt. states they are nervous and would like "the gas".

Medical History:

Medical Hx was reviewed. Pt states she completed the round of Amoxicillin 250 mg bid given at last appointment on 4/11/23. No further changes to medical history since the last visit.

O

OBJECTIVE FINDINGS

Vitals:

BP: 115/80   Pulse: 70   Temp: 98

Clinical Exam

Radiographs:

Preoperative radiograph, progress radiographs, and post-procedural radiograph taken.

Extraoral Exam:

No facial swelling or asymmetry was noted.

Intraoral Exam:

Deep decay on distal of tooth #5. Moderate pain with percussion. Periapical radiolucency noted on tooth #5. No response to cold test.

Pulp Vitality Test

A

ASSESSMENT

N20 required to help mitigate patient anxiety.

Periodontal Condition:

No periodontal defects noted.

Endodontic Condition:

Necrotic pulp with controlled infection

Hard tissue condition:

Missing DO filling with large recurrent decay on tooth #5.

P

PLAN

Endodontic therapy, premolar tooth #5

Treatment rendered today:

The procedure was explained. Alternatives and risks were discussed. Pt. had no questions and consented to treatment.

N2O-given at 40%. Started at 11:15 AM. Stopped at 12:10 PM.

Topical anesthetic placed. 1 carpule of Numbocaine 4% 1:100,000 with epi injected using a 30- gauge short needle into buccal vestibule above tooth #5. Aspiration was negative.

1 carpule of Numbocaine 4% 1:100,000 with epi injected using a 30- gauge short needle intrapulpal.

The patient tolerated the injections and had no adverse reactions. Anesthesia was achieved.

Tooth isolated with rubber dam. Decay removed and chamber accessed.

Two canals found. Buccal canal WL: 20 mm, lingual canal WL: 21 mm - verified with apex locator and radiograph.

Established and maintained patency using crown down technique with rotary files. Copious hypochlorite irrigation, EDTA, and RC prep were used.

Verified placement w/ x-ray, final rinse, dried canals w/ paper points. Filled w/ EndoFiller and gutta percha. Access closed with flowable resin and tooth taken out of occlusion.

Prognosis of the tooth was good.

100% O2 given for 5 minutes. Pt's mental, physical, and emotional condition returned to normal prior to dismissal.

Pt tolerated treatment well.

Post-op instructions were given. Pt was advised the injection site may be sore for a few days. Pt advised not to chew until the anesthetic has worn off but can drink liquids. Pt should stick to a soft diet and avoid chewing on that side until a permanent restoration can be placed.

Rx:

Prescriptions were given for pain management.

Ibuprofen 600mg #30
1 tab every 4-6 hours prn pain

Next visit:

Buildup and crown on #5.

Assistant: A. Helper
Treating Dentist: N. Doh

8

Implant restorations have been around for a long time, but have become more prevalent in general dentistry in recent years. Proper documentation of implant restorations is a crucial part of the procedure. Include the following:

- Date of procedure
- Medical history was reviewed, signed and dated
- Patient's vital signs (pre and post op)
- Consent form signed
- Any issues the patient may be experiencing in that area
- Procedure performed
- Any medications or pre-medications taken
- Type and amount of anesthetic used
- Material used; surgical guides, key and size, drill size
- Bone graft name and type and membrane placed (when applicable)
- Type of Implant, serial number, lot number and any information given about the implant from the manufacturer
- Any new radiographs, cone beam or intra-oral pictures taken
- Post care instructions given
- Post medications given (where applicable)
- Any complications that occurred or the fact that none occurred
- Next visit recommendations

IMPLANT SERVICES S.O.A.P. EXAMPLE

Implant Placement / Date: 1/16/2023 **Time:** 9:30 AM **Dr:** M. Plant

SUBJECTIVE FINDINGS ⊢————————————————————— S

Reason For Visit/Chief Complaint:

The patient, a 55 y.o. male, presents for implant placement #19 accompanied by his wife.

Medical History:

Reviewed medical history. No change since last visit. Pt has an artificial heart valve and requires premedication. Pt. was given 2g Amoxicillin 30 min prior to appt per AHA guidelines.

Dental History:

Tooth #19 was extracted at the Oral Surgeon on 6/11/2022. Bone grafting was done at the time of the extraction and OS has cleared pt. for implant placement.

OBJECTIVE FINDINGS

Vitals:

BP: 130/90   Pulse: 70   Temp: 98

Clinical Exam

Radiographs:

CBCT taken on 01/03/2023 showed adequate bone to receive implant and was used to create a custom placement guide.

Extraoral Exam:

No facial swelling or asymmetry was noted.

Intraoral Exam:

Surgical site appeared to have healed well.

ASSESSMENT

N20 required to help mitigate patient anxiety.

Implant placement #19 using previously fabricated implant guide.

PLAN

Treatment rendered today:

The procedure was explained. Alternatives and risks were discussed, including, but not limited to, pain, bleeding, infection, fracture, treatment failure, damage to adjacent teeth, oroantral communication, need for additional surgery, nerve injury, and paresthesia. Pt. had no questions and consented to treatment. Consent form signed.

N2O-given at 40%. Started at 10:10 AM. Stopped at 11:30 AM.

Topical anesthetic was place. 2 carpules of Numbocaine 4% 1:100,000 with epi injected using a 27- gauge long needle IAN. Aspiration was negative.

The patient tolerated the injections and had no adverse reactions. Anesthesia was achieved.

Implant guide placed and pilot drill used to make single entry through tissue into cortical bone passing to trabecular bone.

Implants-R-Us implant size 4 mm placed. Thumb driver used to anchor the implant firmly in place. Verified placement with CBCT. Placed healing cap. Hemostasis achieved. Implant was placed with no complications.

100% O2 given for 5 minutes. Pt's mental, physical, and emotional condition returned to normal prior to dismissal.

Pt tolerated treatment well.

Verbal and written post op instructions were given to the pt and his wife.

Implant information:

System: Implants-R-Us
Size: 4mm
Lot: 12345
Serial: 1A2B3C

Graft/biological materials used:

N/A

Rx:

Prescriptions were given for pain management and to clear up and prevent infection following implant procedures.

Ibuprofen 600mg #20

Take 1 tab every 4-6 hrs prn pain

No refills

Cephalexin 500mg #30

Take 1 tab 3 times a day until gone

Next visit:

Return in 3 mo to evaluate healing.

Assistant : C. Side
Treating Dentist: M. Plant

Charting Fixed Prosthodontic Procedures

Fixed prosthetics involves any prostheses that are cemented in the mouth permanently, such as crowns and bridges. Different types of materials can be used to create these restorations, including metals, porcelain/ceramic, or a combination of the two. When recording fixed prosthodontic procedures, always note:

- Date of procedure
- Medical history was reviewed, signed and dated
- Patient's vital signs (pre and post op)
- Consent form signed
- Any issues the patient may be experiencing in that area
- Procedure performed
- Any medications or pre-medications taken
- Type and amount of anesthetic used

- Material used; bases, liners, bond, filling material, cement used, impression material or denote CAD CAM
- Rubber dam use and clamp size (when applicable)
- Any new radiographs or intra-oral pictures taken
- Lab used for procedure (if in house lab such as CAD CAM, denote material used, lot number, and any information from the manufacturer)
- Lab work order and estimated date of return
- Type of material used to create restoration
- Shade number and brand of shade guide used
- Post care instructions given
- Post medications given (where applicable)
- Any complications that occurred or the fact that none occurred
- Next visit recommendations

FIXED RESTORATION S.O.A.P. NOTE EXAMPLE #1

Crown and Buildup / **Date:** 4/23/2023 **Time:** 11:00 AM **Dr:** S. Thetic

SUBJECTIVE FINDINGS — S

Reason For Visit/Chief Complaint:

The patient, a 60 y.o. female, presents for buildup and crown on tooth #14. Pt. states they are nervous and would like "the gas".

Medical History:

Medical Hx was reviewed. Pt states she is on new blood pressure medication (LoPress 100mg one tab bid) as of last month.

No further changes to medical history since the last visit.

OBJECTIVE FINDINGS — O

Vitals:

BP: 120/80
Pulse: 80
Temp: 98

Clinical Exam:

Radiographs:

Preoperative radiograph was taken at previous appointment. No further radiographs required.

Extraoral Exam:

No facial swelling or asymmetry was noted.

Intraoral Exam:

Preoperative intraoral photos taken to document decay.

ASSESSMENT — A

N20 required to help mitigate patient anxiety.

Periodontal Condition:

No periodontal defects noted.

Endodontic Condition:

No pain with percussion. No periapical pathology noted.

Hard tissue condition:

Recurrent decay was noted around a large amalgam filling on tooth # 14. Dr. felt inadequate tooth structure would remain to provide sufficient longevity for anything other than full cuspal coverage with a laboratory-processed restoration.

A core buildup was deemed likely due to the size of the existing restoration and decay.

PLAN — P

Buildup and all-porcelain crown on tooth #14.

Treatment rendered today:

The procedure was explained. Alternatives and risks were discussed. Pt. had no questions and consented to treatment.

N2O-given at 40%. Started at 10:15 AM. Stopped at 10:52 AM.

Topical anesthetic placed. 1 carpule of Numbocaine 4% 1:100,000 with epi injected using a 30- gauge short needle into buccal vestibule above tooth #14. Aspiration was negative.

The patient tolerated the injections and had no adverse reactions. Anesthesia was achieved.

A pre-op heavy body double bite was taken.

The large existing amalgam restoration and surrounding decay were removed. A core buildup was necessary for the retention of the crown. 60% of the tooth was removed after full preparation and caries removal, including removal of the entire mesial lingual cusp (see intraoral photo).

The tooth was prepared with SelfEtching Bond 2 and buildup placed using CoreBU XL. Prep was completed with adequate clearance and defined margins. Final impression taken with MadeUP heavy body polyvinyl with a light body wash in a triple tray. Goodtemp temporary cemented with TemporaryBond Clear.

Shade A2. Impressions with signed and dated lab prescription was sent to DentCo Lab.

100% O2 given for 5 minutes. Pt's mental, physical, and emotional condition returned to normal prior to dismissal.

Pt tolerated treatment well.

Post-op instructions were given. Patient advised injection site may be sore for a few days. Pt advised not to chew until the anesthetic has worn off but can drink liquids. Pt should stick to a soft diet and avoid sticky foods. If their bite feels high or if they experience pain or more than slight cold sensitivity they should call the office.

Rx:

No prescriptions given.

Next visit:

Cement permanent crown #14.

Assistant: C. Side
Treating Dentist: S. Thetic

Fixed partial denture (bridge) / **Date:** 02/03/2023 **Time:** 2:00 PM **Dr:** S. Thetic

SUBJECTIVE FINDINGS

Reason For Visit/Chief Complaint:

The patient, a 45 y.o. female, presents for fixed partial denture on upper right.

Medical History:

Medical Hx was reviewed. No changes to medical history since the last visit.

Dental History:

Tooth #4 was extracted in our office on 10/16/2022.

OBJECTIVE FINDINGS

Vitals:

BP: 130/90
Pulse: 70
Temp: 98

At previous visit BP was 130/88. Today Dr. S. Thetic referred pt. to her primary care physician for evaluation of blood pressure.

Clinical Exam

Radiographs: Pre-operative radiographs were taken at previous appointment. No further radiographs required.

Extraoral Exam: No facial swelling or asymmetry was noted.

Intraoral Exam: Extraction site of tooth #4 healed. Ridge appears healthy at site.

Preoperative intraoral photos taken to document missing tooth and restorations on teeth #3 and #5.

ASSESSMENT

Periodontal Condition: Periodontal status of abutment teeth is good. Minimal recession and no active disease noted.

Endodontic Condition: No pain with percussion. No periapical pathology noted.

Hard tissue condition: Abutment teeth are without pathology. Tooth #3 has large MO composite restoration with no signs of recurrent decay.

The alternative of an implant at the site or #4 was discussed. Pt chose to proceed with FPD.

PLAN

Fixed partial denture teeth #3-#5 to replace missing tooth #4 previously extracted.

Treatment rendered today:
The procedure was explained. Alternatives and risks were discussed. Pt. had no questions and consented to treatment.

Topical anesthetic placed. 2 carpules of Numbocaine 4% 1:100,000 with epi injected using a 30- gauge short needle into buccal vestibule above teeth #3 and #5. Aspiration was negative.

The patient tolerated the injections and had no adverse reactions.

Anesthesia was achieved.

A pre-op heavy body double bite was taken.

Prep was completed with adequate clearance and defined margins. Final impression taken with MadeUP heavy body polyvinyl with a light body wash in a triple tray. Goodtemp temporarily cemented with TemporaryBond Clear.

Shade A2. Impressions with signed and dated lab prescriptions were sent to DentCo Lab.

Pt tolerated treatment well.

Post-op instructions were given.

Patient advised injection site may be sore for a few days. Pt advised not to chew until the anesthetic has worn off but can drink liquids. Pt should stick to a soft diet and avoid sticky foods. If their bite feels high or if they experience pain or more than slight cold sensitivity they should call the office.

Rx: No prescriptions given.

Next visit: Cement permanent bridge #3-#5.

Assistant: C. Side
Treating Dentist: S. Thetic

Notes

Notes

_____

_____

_____

_____

_____

_____

_____

_____

_____

_____

_____

_____

_____

_____

Charting Removable Prosthodontic Procedures

A removable prosthesis refers to any restoration a patient can take out of the mouth themselves, such as partial or complete dentures. Always note medical history was reviewed at the appointment. Most patients coming to us for this procedure tend to be elderly and any visit to the dentist can be stressful. Noting their medical history to learn about possible medical conditions is essential even though we are not administering medication. Include the following:

- Date of procedure
- Medical history was reviewed, signed and dated
- Patient's vital signs (pre and post op)
- Consent form signed
- Any issues the patient may be experiencing
- Procedure performed
- Any medications or pre-medications taken
- Measurements taken; midline, canine eminence, lip resting and lip smiling, any other measurements asked of the lab or your doctor
- Material used; impression material, wax rims
- Shade and brand of shade guide
- Lab work order: name of lab and estimated date of return
- Post care instructions given
- Post medications given (where applicable)
- Any complications that occurred or the fact that none occurred
- Next visit recommendations

Complete Denture / **Date:** 4/23/2023 **Time:** 1:00 PM **Dr:** W. Rims

SUBJECTIVE FINDINGS ⊢————————————————————— S

Reason For Visit/Chief Complaint:

The patient, a 71 y.o. male, presented for complete upper denture impressions.

Medical History:

Reviewed medical history. No change since last visit.

Dental History:

Pt. is edentulous in the maxillary and has lower partial denture. He had an existing upper denture done seven years ago at a different provider, which is ill-fitting and unsatisfactory.

OBJECTIVE FINDINGS ⊢————————————————————— O

Vitals:

BP: 140/90
Pulse: 90
Temp: 98

Clinical Exam:

Radiographs:

Panographic radiograph taken on 2/14/2023. No new radiographs.

Current denture is 7 years old. The teeth are worn and tooth #7 is broken. New denture is recommended due to loss of vertical dimension and ill fit.

ASSESSMENT ⊢————————————————————— A

Pt. needs new maxillary denture. Reviewed alternate treatment plan of implant supported FPD or hybrid prosthesis, but pt chose to continue with removable complete denture.

PLAN ⊢————————————————————— P

Maxillary complete denture

Treatment rendered today:
Full arch impressions were taken of maxillary using polysulfide rubber impression material. Mandibular full arch impression was taken using alginate and bite registration established.

Tooth shade A2. Signed and dated lab slip sent to DentCo Lab for fabrication of wax try-in.

Rx:
No prescriptions given.

Next visit:
Wax try in

Assistant: M. Pression
Treating Dentist: W. Rims

Charting Oral and Maxillofacial Surgical Procedures

The scope of oral and maxillofacial surgical procedures is vast and there are many complex procedures that can fall under this category. Record each procedure thoroughly and accurately in order to capture the best information on what has taken place at each visit. Include the following:

- Date of procedure
- Medical history was reviewed, signed and dated
- Patient's vital signs (pre and post op)
- Consent form signed
- Any issues the patient may be experiencing in that area
- Procedure performed
- Any medications or pre-medications taken
- Type and amount of anesthetic used
- Any dressings, or packings placed
- Sutures, type of suture or the lack thereof
- Post care instructions given
- Post medications given (where applicable)
- Any complications that occurred or the fact that none occurred
- Next visit recommendations

Accurate Reporting of Biopsies

Stedman's Medical Dictionary defines a biopsy as the "removal and examination, usually microscopic, of tissue from the living body, often to determine whether a tumor is malignant or benign; biopsies are also done for diagnosis of disease processes such as infections." The term may be used to describe either the procedure being performed, or the sample of tissue obtained. Biopsy procedures performed in a dental practice are primarily classified as either incisional or excisional. Also, a specimen may be obtained by collecting cells from the mucosa.

Incisional Biopsy

In an incisional biopsy, a small sample of tissue is taken from a suspicious lesion. This sample may be of a soft tissue lesion or hard or osseous lesion. This tissue is then sent to a pathology laboratory for microscopic examination. Based on the pathologist's report, additional surgery may be scheduled for definitive treatment to remove the lesion.

The sample may be taken using a scalpel, a punch instrument, or a laser. The method used to obtain the specimen is not relevant to the procedure code reported or the fee charged. An additional fee may not be billed to the payor or the patient for the use of a laser.

Excisional biopsy

Excisional biopsies involve the removal of an entire lesion. This may be performed as definitive treatment following a previous incisional biopsy or as an initial procedure. Tissue removed during the procedure is often sent to a pathology lab for examination. Tissue removal is a component of the procedure; therefore, an additional biopsy procedure is not reported separately for the same lesion on the same date of service.

When reporting a biopsy to a medical payor, the procedure code reported is based on the anatomical location of the lesion. Therefore, there are many procedure codes from which to choose. Applicable dental codes are based on the size of the lesion, the complexity of the biopsy procedure, and whether the lesion is benign or malignant. Dental payors rarely reimburse these procedures, as most are covered by medical insurance.

Anytime a specimen is sent for microscopic examination, it is advisable to hold the claim until the pathology report is received. The pathologist will assign a diagnosis code based on the findings. This code should be reported on the claim as the primary diagnosis. Holding a claim for the pathology report is important, not only because it is the most accurate diagnosis, but also because this diagnosis will be a permanent part of the patient's clinical record. It is inaccurate to report a lesion as malignant based solely on visual findings. Conversely, if a lesion is reported to an insurance payor as benign, it may be difficult to support the necessity of additional treatment if the pathology report indicates malignancy.

There may be times, however, when the provider determines a lesion is benign and no pathology examination is required. Even when no pathology report is available, medical payors will still require a diagnosis code.

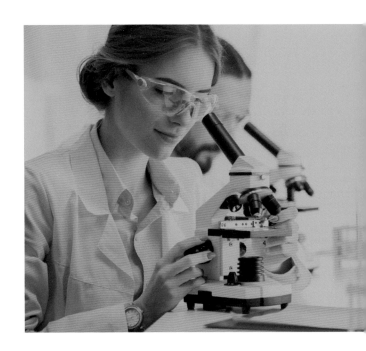

ORAL & MAXILLOFACIAL SURGERY S.O.A.P EXAMPLES

Simple extraction / **Date:** 4/23/2023 **Time:** 1:30 PM **Dr:** I. Pullem

SUBJECTIVE FINDINGS ───────────────────── S

Reason For Visit/Chief Complaint:
The patient, a 22 y.o. male, presents for extraction of tooth #1 due to pain from eruption, accompanied by his wife.

Medical History:
Medical Hx was reviewed. No changes to medical history since the last visit.

Dental History:
Pt. has had pain in area of tooth #1 that has been keeping him up at night.

Social History:
Pt. is a 1 pack/week smoker.

OBJECTIVE FINDINGS   O

Vitals:

BP: 120/80
Pulse: 80
Temp: 98
Blood Glucose Level: 120

Clinical Exam:

Radiographs:

Panographic radiograph and PA taken at last appointment on 4/10/2023. No further radiographs required.

Extraoral Exam:

No facial swelling or asymmetry was noted. No tenderness on palpation on the face, neck, or jaw joints.

No pain or crepitus was noted with jaw movements in TMJ evaluation.

Intraoral Exam:

Inflamed and swollen tissue around partially erupted tooth #1. Painful to the touch.

ASSESSMENT   A

Periodontal Condition: Pericoronitis around tooth #1

PLAN   P

Extraction of tooth #1

Treatment rendered today:

The procedure was explained. Alternatives and risks were discussed, including, but not limited to, pain, bleeding, infection, fracture, treatment failure, damage to adjacent teeth, oroantral communication, need for additional surgery, nerve injury, and paresthesia. Pt. had no questions and consented to treatment. Consent form signed.

Topical anesthetic placed. 1 carpule of Numbocaine 4% 1:100,000 with epi injected using a 30- gauge short needle into buccal vestibule above tooth #1. Aspiration was negative. Half carpule of Numbocaine 4% 1:100,000 with epi injected using a 30- gauge short needle into palatal tissue.

The patient tolerated the injections and had no adverse reactions. Anesthesia was achieved.

Gingiva was retracted and the tooth elevated using a straight elevator. Tooth was removed without incident using forceps.

Hemostasis was achieved using gauze and pressure.

Pt tolerated treatment well.

Verbal and written post-operative instructions were given to the patient and his wife.

Rx:

Prescriptions were given for pain management.

Ibuprofen 600mg #20

Take 1 tab every 4-6 hrs prn pain

No refills

Next visit:

Assistant: I. Care
Treating Dentist: I. Pullem

Notes

8

Notes

Charting Orthodontic Procedures

Today's orthodontics offer a wide range of services. From traditional bands and brackets to aligners and ortho appliances, orthodontic services encompass many different procedures. Items that should be noted in the clinical record include:

- Date of procedure

- Medical history was reviewed, signed and dated

- Consent form signed

- Any issues the patient may be experiencing

- Orthodontic records;

  - Intraoral Images

  - Panoramic X-Ray

  - Cephalometric film

  - Impressions/CAD CAM Scan

  - Bite registration

  - Type of orthodontic services chosen (i.e.; Bands and Brackets vs. Aligners vs. Appliances)

  - Limited or comprehensive orthodontic plan

- Lab work order (where applicable)

- Post care instructions given

- Any complications that occurred or the fact that none occurred

- Next visit recommendations

Comprehensive Adult Ortho / **Date:** 4/23/2023 **Time:** 9:00 AM **Dr:** M. Straighten

SUBJECTIVE FINDINGS

Reason For Visit/Chief Complaint:

The patient, a 19 y.o. female, presents for ortho evaluation and records.

Medical History:

Medical Hx was reviewed. No changes to medical history since the last visit

Dental History:

Pt. was last seen in our office for recare on 02/03/23. No outstanding treatment needs prior to orthodontics.

OBJECTIVE FINDINGS

Vitals:

BP: 110/75
Pulse: 70
Temp: 98

Clinical Exam:

Radiographs:

Panoramic and cephalometric radiographs were taken.

Extraoral Exam:

Facial and profile photos were taken for orthodontic records.

Intraoral Exam:

Maxillary anterior teeth are proclined and pt has an overjet of 5 mm.

ASSESSMENT

Class II Division 1 retrognathic.

PLAN

Comprehensive adult orthodontic treatment using traditional brackets

Treatment rendered today:

The procedure was explained. Alternatives and risks were discussed. Pt. had no questions and consented to treatment. A consent form was signed.

Panoramic and cephalometric radiographs were taken.

Using retractors and mirrors, intraoral photos were taken from the anterior and both sides in occlusion. Extraoral photos of full face and profile were also taken.

Alginate impressions were taken to create diagnostic models of the maxillary and mandibular arches.

Rx:

No prescriptions given.

Next visit:

Band and bracket placement

Assistant: M. Pression
Treating Dentist: M. Straighten

Notes

_____

_____

_____

_____

_____

_____

_____

_____

_____

_____

_____

_____

Charting Adjunctive Services

Adjunctive general services such as occlusal guards have become more popular in today's dentistry due to extensive restorative work. Such general services are just as important as any other service when it comes to documentation. Include the following in your report:

- Date of procedure
- Date of procedure
- Medical history was reviewed, signed and dated
- Patient's vital signs (pre and post op)
- Consent form signed
- Any issues the patient may be experiencing
- Procedure performed
- Lab work order
- Any new radiographs or intra-oral pictures taken
- Post care instructions given
- Any complications that occurred or the fact that none occurred
- Next visit recommendations ıll

Date: 4/23/2023 **Time:** 3:30 PM **Dr:** B. Rux

SUBJECTIVE FINDINGS — S

Reason For Visit/Chief Complaint:

The patient, a 47 y.o. male, presents for impressions for a lower night guard.

Medical History:

Medical Hx was reviewed. No changes to medical history since the last visit.

Dental History:

Pt. has hx of bruxism with obvious wear on posterior teeth. Pt received new anterior porcelain crowns on 04/19/23.

OBJECTIVE FINDINGS — O

Vitals:
BP: 120/80
Pulse: 80
Temp: 98

Clinical Exam:

Radiographs:

No new radiographs necessary.

Extraoral Exam:

No facial swelling or asymmetry was noted. No tenderness on palpation on the face, neck, or jaw joints.

No pain or crepitus was noted with jaw movements in TMJ evaluation.

Intraoral Exam:

Wear facets obvious on posterior occlusal surfaces.

ASSESSMENT — A

Hard mandibular occlusal guard advised to protect teeth including new anterior porcelain restorations.

PLAN — P

Occlusal guard —
hard appliance, full arch

Treatment rendered today:

Full arch alginate impressions were taken of maxillary and mandibular. Bite registration taken. Stone models created.

Signed and dated lab slip sent to DentCo Lab for fabrication of lower acrylic night guard.

Rx:

No prescriptions given.

Next visit:

Occlusal guard delivery

Assistant: I. Grind
Treating Dentist: B. Rux

Dental practitioners classify patients' periodontal health based on a specific classification system. A new classification system was adopted and endorsed at the 2017 World Workshop on the Classification of Periodontal and Peri-Implant Diseases and Conditions.

CHAPTER NINE

Documenting for Periodontics

Perio Classification System

Dental practitioners classify patients' periodontal health based on a specific classification system. A new classification system was adopted and endorsed at the 2017 World Workshop on the Classification of Periodontal and Peri-Implant Diseases and Conditions. This event was co-hosted by the American Academy of Periodontology (AAP) and the European Federation of Periodontology (EFP).

This is the first update to the classification system since 1999. This system enables clinicians to form a more robust diagnosis of the patient's periodontal condition and to establish appropriate treatment plans to manage it. The updated classification system also improves the documentation and submission process.

Categories of Periodontal Diseases and Conditions

As detailed in the Journal of Clinical Periodontology, the new classification system identifies three types of periodontal diseases and conditions and features several important subcategories.

1. Periodontal Health, Gingival Diseases, and Conditions. Includes periodontal and gingival health, gingivitis related to dental biofilm, and gingival diseases or conditions not related to biofilm.

2. Periodontitis. Necrotizing periodontal diseases, periodontitis (no longer identified as chronic or aggressive), and periodontitis as a manifestation of systemic diseases.

3. Other Conditions Affecting the Periodontium. Systemic diseases affecting the periodontium, periodontal abscesses or endodontic-periodontal lesions, mucogingival deformities and conditions, traumatic occlusal forces, and tooth and prosthesis-related factors.

Staging and Grading System

The new classification system has two key components: identifying (1) a stage and (2) a grade of periodontal disease involvement for the patient. The AAP reports that this new system "provides a structure for treatment planning and for monitoring a patient's response to therapy."

Stages

Stages indicate the severity of the disease at presentation and the complexity of disease management, according to the Journal of Periodontology. The stages range from Stage I to Stage IV, with the lowest number representing the least severe form of the disease. The stage of the condition is determined by a variety of factors, including the amount of clinical attachment loss, the percentage of radiographic bone loss around the tooth, the number of teeth lost due to periodontal disease, probing depth, and the complexity of treatment.

Grades

Grades provide supplemental information about the biologic features of periodontitis and incorporate a history based analysis of the rate of periodontal progression. Grading includes the risk of further progression, the potential poor outcomes, and the risk that the disease or its treatment may negatively affect the general health of the patient. The three grades are: **A:** Slow progression; **B:** Moderate progression; **C:** Rapid progression.

Grades are based on clinical attachment level and/or radiographic bone loss, percentage of bone loss, and case phenotype (determined by the body's reaction to the presence of biofilm). The grading system also considers smoking and hyperglycemia in diabetes as individual risk factors.

Categories of Peri-Implant Diseases and Conditions

Due to the growing number of patients receiving implants, it was necessary to integrate information about implant complications. The new system also includes four new categories for peri-implant conditions and diseases.

1. **Peri-implant health.** A lack of visible inflammation. No bleeding upon probing. Consider code D1110 or D4910 (natural teeth must be present); or D6080 for maintenance of implant supported fixed prothesis.

2. **Peri-implant mucositis.** Visible signs of inflammation. Bleeding on probing. Consider code D6081.

3. **Peri-implantitis.** Inflammation of peri-implant mucosa followed by progressive loss of surrounding bone. Consider code D6101 or D6102 and/or any additional services to treat the bone loss.

4. **Hard and soft tissue implant site deficiencies.** Deficiencies of the alveolar ridge caused by natural healing, extraction trauma, infections, or a variety of other factors affecting hard and soft tissue. Report any surgical services necessary to treat the deficiencies.

Impact on Patient Care

As explained by the AAP, this new classification system will help clinicians develop an appropriate treatment plan strategy based on a patient's specific needs. This system enables dental professionals to individualize patient treatment more comprehensively by providing significantly more diagnostic, targeted treatment details than the previous classification system.

The new periodontitis classification system may also help in discussions regarding health behaviors and conditions with patients. Using these categories and stages while explaining the expected progression of periodontal disease with a patient will hopefully motivate them to improve modifiable risk factors, such as A1C levels for diabetics or to stop other risk factors like cigarette smoking.

A more detailed periodontal and peri-implant diseases and conditions classification scheme will also allow the integration of risk factors, like smoking and the body's response to biofilm, into the patient's periodontal diagnosis and potential disease progression. This could also help patients link their oral health with their overall health.

Conclusion

This new classification system utilizes specific classifications of diseases, coupled with a staging and grading system. This improvement in documentation allows the dentist and hygienist to individualize patient periodontal care and address multi-dimensional factors. The overall goal is to improve treatment outcomes in patients' oral health. For more information visit https://sites.perio.org/wp-content/uploads/2019/08/Staging-and-Grading-Periodontitis.pdf

Periodontal Re-Evaluation

Periodontal therapy makes up a large part of the hygiene service mix of many general dental practices. Therefore, one of the most common periodontal coding questions asked is "What code reports a six week re-evaluation visit following scaling and root planing?" Unfortunately, there is not a universal answer. Rather, the answer varies depending on the procedure(s) performed. Also, the procedure(s) performed are dependent on your practice's specific protocols and the doctor's recommendation(s). Below, several possible coding scenarios are outlined for reporting a periodontal re-evaluation visit.

D1110, prophylaxis – adult, may be reported when a prophylaxis is performed at the periodontal re-evaluation visit in support of good periodontal health. This procedure typically has a good chance of reimbursement.

Bear in mind that a few plans may cancel the patient's periodontal benefit if a prophylaxis is performed after scaling and root planing, prior to periodontal maintenance. Some plans have a frequency limitation of 30 to 60 days between any scaling and root planing procedure and a prophylaxis procedure, regardless of the order performed. This is plan-specific. Be sure to verify the patient's benefits prior to initiating this treatment sequence. Furthermore, review any Preferred Provider Organization (PPO) contracts and Processing Policy Manuals for frequency limitations regarding reporting a prophylaxis following scaling and root planing.

Examples of contract language that may be found in the Processing Policy Manual are:

- "A separate fee for all necessary postoperative care, finishing procedures (D1110, D1120, D4341, D4342, D4355, D4910), evaluations, or other surgical procedures (except soft tissue grafts) on the same date of service or for three months following the initial periodontal therapy by the same dentist/dental office is non-billable."

- "The fee for the following services: D1110, D1120, D4355, and/or D4910 will be non-billable if the services are rendered by the same dentist/dental office within 30 days after the most recent scaling and root planing (D4341, D4342) or other periodontal therapy."

PPO contract verbiage can differ widely among payors, so it is imperative to read all of your current PPO Processing Policy Manuals for each PPO in which your practice participates. Additionally processing policy provisions can and will be changed from time to time, as long as proper written notification is provided, as outlined in your PPO contract.

D0180, comprehensive periodontal evaluation – new or established patient, may be reported if the dentist performed the oral evaluation and performed a complete periodontal probing and charting for patients with periodontal disease or who are at greater risk for developing periodontal disease. A complete periodontal charting and probing includes, but is not limited to, six-point probing depths per tooth, bleeding points, clinical attachment loss (CAL), areas of furcation involvement, mobility, recession, etc.

As with all oral evaluations, a dentist must perform the oral evaluation. A dental team member may collect information (e.g., take radiographs, periodontal probing, charting, etc.), but the dentist is the only one who can make a diagnosis. (Exception – a few states now allow hygienists to make a diagnosis. A properly licensed independent hygienist practicing within the scope of practice in certain states may be allowed to diagnose but only in specific states that permit it.)

D0180 shares a frequency limitation with other evaluations, such as D0120, D0140, and D0150. Some dental plans may remap D0180 to D0120 for reimbursement. A PPO may also disallow the difference in the allowed amount of D0180 and D0120 unless the D0180 is the initial oral evaluation performed by the dentist providing the periodontal maintenance therapy.

D0171, re-evaluation – postoperative office visit, may be reported if the dentist performed the oral evaluation and needs to re-evaluate the patient after an operative service. The payor may deny reimbursement, as many plans consider post-operative care inclusive in the global fee for the procedure when performed within a predetermined time period, as established in the dental plan document. If D0171 is reimbursed, it may be paid at a lower rate than D0180. Thus, this code is not recommended.

D4999, unspecified periodontal procedure, by report, may be reported if the patient is only seen by a hygienist, no evaluation is performed by the doctor, and periodontal probing and charting is performed to determine the tissue response to periodontal treatment. There is not a separate code to report periodontal probing and charting. Typically D4999 is not reimbursed.

D4381, localized delivery of antimicrobial agents via controlled release vehicle into diseased cervicular tissue, per tooth, may be reported when Arestin®, Atridox®, or Periochip®, etc. is indicated and placed at the re-evaluation appointment.

Coverage for D4381 varies greatly among dental plans and should be verified prior to initiating treatment. Reimbursement may be considered when placed at the re-evaluation visit following scaling and root planing. However, many dental plans exclude reimbursement if the antimicrobial agent is placed on the same date of service as scaling and root planing. Payors may consider reimbursement when the agent is placed at a visit following active periodontal therapy in unresolved sites of infection (bleeding on probing), which indicates active disease.

D4381 is reported on a per tooth basis, regardless of the number of sites treated per tooth. Attach a narrative to the claim that identifies each site treated. The fee per tooth may reflect the number of sites treated. It is acceptable to have more than one fee for the same procedure, as long as all patients are treated the same in similar circumstances. For example, the fee for one site per tooth may be $30, the fee for two sites per tooth $50, the fee for three sites per tooth $70, and so on. However, if you are in-network, the negotiated fee for D4381 will remain the same, regardless of the number of sites treated around the tooth.

A periodontal charting and probing, as well as radiographs should be attached to the claim to support the necessity of D4381. Also include the diagnosis in the narrative.

D4381 includes both the furnishing of the agent and placement. The patient's medical pharmacy benefits may possibly be available through a specialized pharmacy to cover the cost of the agent. Reach out to the manufacturer's representative for information regarding pharmacy programs. In this case, the dentist reports D4381 for placement of the agent and should consider a reduced fee when reporting the placement only.

D4910, periodontal maintenance, if performed, may be reported at the six week re-evaluation visit. While D4910 describes the service, it is not typically reimbursed unless it is performed at least 90 days following completion of active periodontal therapy (SRP, gingival flap surgery, osseous surgery). Some PPOs will disallow the charge for D4910 if performed within 90 days of active periodontal therapy.

D4910 includes a prophylaxis and site specific scaling and root planing, where indicated. The clinical documentation should reflect that a prophylaxis was performed as part of the periodontal maintenance procedure, and the areas of site specific scaling and root planing should be noted. Note that D4910 and prophylaxis (D1110) now includes cleaning any implant crowns, along with the natural dentition.

Frequency limitations vary by dental plan for D4910. In instances where D4910 benefits are denied due to frequency, appeal the denial and request an alternate benefit of D1110. Include a narrative stating, "If periodontal maintenance benefits are not available, please consider an alternate benefit of a prophylaxis (D1110), as a prophylaxis was performed as part of the periodontal maintenance procedure." Remember, only the information included in the chart note may be included in a narrative attached to a claim. Again, keep in mind a few payors may cancel the patient's periodontal benefits if a prophylaxis is paid.

While the most common procedures performed at a re-evaluation visit have been noted, these may not align with your treatment performed. Remember—always report what you do, regardless of insurance benefits or lack thereof. Be specific and thorough with documentation to support all treatments performed, including the diagnosis. Dental plan benefits vary greatly among payors and should be verified prior to starting treatment. If you are an in-network provider, you should carefully review all PPO Processing Policy Manuals for provisions applicable to the periodontal codes discussed above.

Guide to Reporting D4346

For years, there has been a continuing debate on how to properly report a treatment that is more complex than a prophylaxis ("prophy"), but does not qualify as scaling and root planing ("SRP") because there is no bone loss. When a patient has moderate or severe gingival inflammation, but no bone loss, this procedure requires more time and effort to complete than a standard prophy. Thus D4346 was added to CDT in 2017.

D4346 Scaling in presence of generalized moderate or severe gingival inflammation – full mouth, after oral evaluation

The removal of plaque, calculus and stains from supra- and subgingival tooth surfaces when there is generalized moderate or severe gingival inflammation in the absence of periodontitis. It is indicated for patients who have swollen, inflamed gingiva, generalized suprabony pockets, and moderate to severe bleeding on probing. Should not be reported in conjunction with prophylaxis, scaling and root planing, or debridement procedures.

The Code's Purpose

Why was a scaling code needed? Before D4346 was added, there were CDT codes to report procedures for patients with a generally healthy periodontium or patients with periodontal disease and accompanying attachment loss (e.g., periodontal pockets and bone loss). However, there were no codes to describe the treatment of moderate or severe gingivitis (inflammation).

Thus, there was need for a code to report the therapeutic treatment of patients with generalized moderate or severe gingival inflammation, with or without pseudo-pockets, but exhibiting no bone loss. The objective of adding code D4346 is to provide more accurate documentation of the services performed for patients with moderate or severe generalized inflammation.

In the past, D1110 (prophylaxis) would have been reported to describe a scaling procedure performed on a patient with a documented diagnosis of generalized moderate or severe gingival inflammation. This scaling procedure was often wrongly upcoded to a scaling and root planing procedure. The addition of D4346 closed this gap, allowing more accurate and appropriate documentation and reporting of the procedure.

Prior to the addition of D4346, this procedure was sometimes referred to as a "difficult prophy" because of the degree of difficulty and time taken to perform the procedure. However, coding for a prophylaxis is not based on the difficulty of the procedure or the time taken to perform the prophylaxis. The prophylaxis fee could be adjusted to reflect the degree of difficulty and additional time needed.

Code D4346 does not define a "difficult prophylaxis" and should not be reported as such. D4346 should be reported for patients with generalized moderate or severe gingival inflammation in the absence of attachment loss. In other words, the procedure is based on the diagnosis, not the required time or difficulty of the treatment.

If a patient presents with heavy plaque, calculus, staining, etc., which requires more time and effort, this "difficult prophy" is accurately reported as D1110 prophylaxis, regardless of the difficulty and/or time needed to complete the procedure.

D4346 is a therapeutic service performed after oral evaluation and diagnosis of gingivitis to remove all deposits and allow tissue healing. An oral evaluation and D4346 may be performed on the same service date.

D4346 is not followed by D4910 (periodontal maintenance). D4346 is performed on patients who do not exhibit a loss of attachment. D4910 is a recare procedure that includes site specific root planing as needed on patients who have been treated for significant attachment loss. D4910 follows active periodontal therapy.

Code D4346 was assigned to the Code's periodontics category rather than the prevention section. Why would a procedure for "scaling in the presence of...generalized gingival inflammation" performed for a patient who does not have periodontal disease, but has inflammation (gingivitis), be assigned to the periodontics category?

The procedure is considered *therapeutic* for a patient in a diseased state, as noted by this sentence in the D4346 descriptor: "It is indicated for patients who have swollen, inflamed gingiva, generalized suprabony pockets, and moderate to severe bleeding on probing." When a patient

is diagnosed with *generalized* gingivitis following an oral evaluation, this scaling procedure treats the generalized gingival inflammation and pseudo pockets present.

Proper Reporting

Documentation is important in supporting the treatment and obtaining reimbursement of D4346 and subsequent gingival treatments. Documentation should include periodontal charting that records pocket depths and bleeding on probing. Photographs, radiographs, and other diagnostic images are particularly helpful to document the gingiva's condition (e.g., visible localized or generalized inflammation) or to demonstrate the absence of bone loss. These images will prove useful to answer questions that may arise in the reimbursement process.

D4346 is a full mouth procedure that is typically completed on a single service date, often at the first visit to the practice. However, patient comfort and acceptance may require the procedure to be provided over multiple appointments. If more than one appointment is required, the date of completion is the date of service.

When scheduling D4346 and subsequent gingival procedures, it is important to wait an acceptable time period between completion of D4346 and delivery of a subsequent prophylaxis as part of the patient's initial preventive regimen. Technically, there is no set waiting period. However, D4346 is a therapeutic procedure to improve the patient's oral health and a reasonable amount of time (typically two to six weeks) should be allowed for healing before the patient can resume a regular preventive regimen that may include oral prophylaxis.

In very limited circumstances, a patient treated with D4346 may subsequently develop periodontitis and need a scaling and root planing procedure following bone loss. D4346 is not necessarily exclusive of D4341 or D4342, as the dentist may recognize progressive, active periodontal disease at a future date.

CDT fully supports the documentation and reporting of procedures at any time the dentist determines they are necessary for the patient's oral health. This is a matter of clinical judgment by the treating dentist. Benefit design should not guide the clinical determination of procedures performed.

Scaling and Root Planing (SRP)

Scaling and root planing (SRP) remains one of the most misunderstood and misused codes in all of CDT. Payors have also suggested that SRP codes have been widely abused. As a result, obtaining reimbursement for scaling and root planing can be challenging for most dental practices. The key to successful adjudication of SRP claims is proper documentation.

Claims may be rejected or denied due to a lack of supporting documentation. The presence of pocket depths is only part of the story.The supporting documentation must include evidence of active disease and radiographic bone loss in order to establish medical necessity.

Scaling and root planing procedures are therapeutic treatments and are indicated for patients with active periodontal disease. Typically, there must be evidence of bleeding on probing indicating active disease, pocket depths of 4-5mm or greater, radiographic evidence of bone loss, and documented clinical attachment loss for SRP to be reimbursed. Root planing includes removal of cementum and dentin that is rough and/or permeated by calculus or contaminated with toxins or microorganisms. Without loss of attachment and exposed root area, root planing is not possible.

Patients with pseudo pocketing, gingival inflammation, and bleeding, but without bone loss and attachment loss, do not qualify for SRP treatment. Furthermore, scaling calculus and bacterial deposits from enamel surfaces, whether supragingival or subgingival, does not constitute SRP. Scaling supragingival and subgingival areas of the anatomical tooth crown is accurately reported as a prophylaxis, D1110 or D4346, as outlined below. Intentionally reporting SRP when there is no evidence of bone loss may be considered upcoding and could be considered fraudulent billing.

For the patient with a diagnosis of moderate to severe gingival inflammation with pocketing, bleeding on probing, and no bone loss or attachment loss, it is appropriate to report D4346. The patient's inflammatory condition may range from acute to chronic, but there are very specific diagnostic criteria to establish moderate or severe gingival inflammation (gingivitis).

Additionally, the descriptor clearly indicates that D4346 cannot be reported in conjunction with D1110 (prophylaxis, adult), D4341 and D4342 (scaling and root planing), or D4355 (full mouth debridement) when performed on the same service date. The subsequent treatment visit, considered part of the initial therapy sequence, would typically be a conventional prophylaxis, D1110. In most cases, appropriate treatment and improved hygiene will reverse the moderate or severe gingival inflammation. The patient would then return for prophylaxis treatment as deemed appropriate by the doctor, typically in six month intervals.

D4346 fills a gap that had been missing in the CDT code set for years. Scaling supragingival and subgingival areas of the tooth crown below the gum line may also be accurately reported as Prophylaxis (D1110). D1110 may be appropriate when the patient has *localized* gingivitis but does not meet the criteria of D4346.

Clinical Attachment Loss (CAL)

Clinical attachment loss occurs as a result of bone loss due to periodontal disease. Some payors may deny SRP claims when clinical attachment loss is not clearly documented on the chart.

The CEJ is the point where the enamel surface meets the cementum surface on the root. If the base of the pocket does not extend below the CEJ, then there is no loss of attachment and root planing cannot be performed.

The amount of CAL, if any, must be clearly documented in the patient's chart.

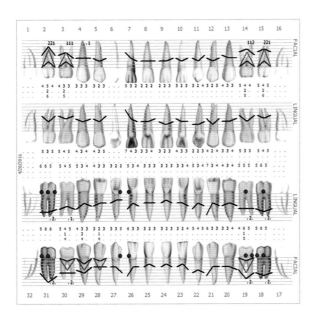

The Clinical Note

The clinical note must be thorough and complete to support a SRP claim. Clinical notes should, at a minimum, include the following:

- Diagnosis of periodontitis (i.e., generalized chronic moderate periodontitis) using the new Staging and Grading of Periodontal Disease will help with diagnosis and payor consideration.

- Description of the periodontal condition (i.e., location of bleeding points, purulent discharge, increase in pocket depths, loss of attachment, recession, mobility, etc.)

- Medical conditions that may be a contributing factor to the patient's periodontal disease (i.e., diabetes, pregnancy, cardiovascular disease, etc.)

- Documentation that both scaling and root planing and polishing were performed and the area(s) treated. (Often, the clinical note will include that scaling was performed but fail to note that root planing was also performed.)

SRP Claim Submission

There are two CDT codes that report SRP, D4341 (periodontal scaling and root planing – four or more teeth per quadrant) and D4342 (periodontal scaling and root planing – one to three teeth per quadrant). The only difference in D4341 and D4342 is the number of teeth in a given quadrant that require SRP. Report the appropriate code and indicate the quadrant treated on the claim form. Many payors require the treated teeth numbers to be listed on the claim form when reporting D4342.

For SRP treatment to be considered for reimbursement, the supporting documentation must include radiographic evidence of bone loss (most payors require a recent full mouth series), clinical periodontal attachment loss, bleeding points, and probing depths. Include the following documentation with the claim submission:

- Full mouth radiographs, that are of diagnostic quality, showing radiographic evidence of bone loss and/or root surface calculus and deposits. Intra-oral – complete series of radiographic images (D0210) is the typical standard of care for diagnosing periodontal disease. Some payors may reject a SRP claim if any other radiographs are submitted as supporting documentation.

- Complete periodontal charting and probing. This should include, but is not limited to, 6 point probing depths, bleeding points, areas of gingival recession, areas of furcation involvement, tooth mobility, CAL, suppuration, etc.

- A narrative that includes the diagnosis, description of the periodontal condition, and any medical conditions that may be a contributing factor. The narrative submitted should mirror the clinical note.

Note: Some payors no longer accept a narrative and will only accept clinical notes for claim adjudication.

Diagnoses Codes

Documentation is key for SRP reimbursement. With some payors already requiring diagnoses codes (ICD-10-CM) to be reported when submitting claims for SRP, it is important that the documentation be thorough to support the diagnosis. The diagnosis must be documented in order for the appropriate ICD-10-CM code to be applied.

ICD-10-CM codes are very specific. When the diagnosis is not clearly noted, an unspecified diagnosis code must be used. Some common primary diagnoses codes that may apply to SRP claims are:

K03.6 Deposits (accretions) on teeth

K05.20 Aggressive periodontitis, unspecified

K05.211 Aggressive periodontitis, localized, slight

K05.212 Aggressive periodontitis, localized, moderate

K05.213 Aggressive periodontitis, localized, severe

K05.221 Aggressive periodontitis, generalized, slight

K05.222 Aggressive periodontitis, generalized, moderate

K05.223 Aggressive periodontitis, generalized, severe

K05.311 Chronic periodontitis, localized, slight

K05.312 Chronic periodontitis, localized, moderate

K05.313 Chronic periodontitis, localized, severe

K05.321 Chronic periodontitis, generalized, slight

K05.322 Chronic periodontitis, generalized, moderate

K05.323 Chronic periodontitis, generalized, severe

K05.6 Periodontal disease, unspecified

Note: Do not report an unspecified code when a more specific code is available.

Additionally, a secondary diagnosis code may be applied to indicate that a condition exists as a contributing factor to the patient's disease (e.g., E11.630, Type 2 diabetes mellitus with periodontal disease). Refer to our book publication *Medical Dental Cross Coding With Confidence 2023* for more information.

Reporting D4910 vs. D1110

Is alternating D4910 (periodontal maintenance) with D1110 (prophylaxis) appropriate? Is reverting from D4910 status to D1110 appropriate?

Alternating periodontal maintenance (D4910) with a prophylaxis (D1110) for the periodontal patient continues to be a controversial topic with various opinions and interpretations. Along with the alternating controversy, there is confusion as to whether a periodontal patient receiving periodontal maintenance (D4910) may be augmented and periodontal health supported with a prophylaxis (D1110).

This chapter discusses the appropriateness of submitting D4910 vs. D1110. We will begin by reviewing the various definitions and interpretations of the codes, then analyze their proper reporting.

CDT 2022 Nomenclatures and Descriptors

D1110 Prophylaxis – adult

Removal of plaque, calculus and stains from the tooth structures and implants in the permanent and transitional dentition. It is intended to control local irritational factors.

D4910 Periodontal maintenance

This procedure is instituted following periodontal therapy and continues at varying intervals, determined by the clinical evaluation of the dentist, for the life of the dentition or any implant replacements. It includes removal of the bacterial plaque and calculus from supragingival and subgingival regions, site specific scaling and root planing where indicated, and polishing the teeth. If new or recurring periodontal disease appears, additional diagnostic and treatment procedures must be considered.

AAP Definitions

"Prophylaxis, oral:

The removal of plaque, calculus, and stains from the exposed and unexposed surfaces of the teeth by scaling and polishing as a preventive measure for the control of local irritational factors."

"Periodontal maintenance (formerly referred to as Supportive Periodontal Therapy [SPT], Preventive Maintenance, Recall Maintenance):

Procedures performed at selected intervals to assist the periodontal patient in maintaining oral health. As part of periodontal therapy, an interval is established for periodic ongoing care. Maintenance procedures are under the supervision of the dentist and typically include an update of the medical and dental histories, radiographic review, extraoral and intraoral soft tissue examination, dental examination, periodontal evaluation, removal of the bacterial flora from crevicular and pocket areas, scaling and root planing where indicated, polishing of the teeth, and a review of the patient's plaque control efficacy. Periodontal maintenance procedures following active therapy is not synonymous with a prophylaxis."

6

Commentary

CDT's definition of a prophylaxis describes a specific clinical procedure. It is listed in CDT as a preventive procedure, but the code itself does not include the words "preventive measure."

Reporting D1110 is always appropriate for patients who do not exhibit signs or symptoms of periodontal disease. However, D1110's nomenclature and descriptor is silent regarding whether the patient is periodontal disease free. The AAP definition of a prophylaxis says it is a "preventive measure." However, a prophylaxis may be performed in an area or areas of the mouth with periodontal disease whether these areas have been treated previously or require periodontal treatment.

Because the CDT definition of a prophylaxis differs from the AAP definition, there is some confusion concerning proper reporting. Always report any dental procedure based on the current CDT nomenclature and descriptor.

D1110 vs. D4910

Periodontal maintenance is appropriate for ongoing maintenance of the periodontal health of patients with a history of active periodontal disease. It is considered a therapeutic treatment and includes site specific scaling and root planing, where indicated. Periodontal maintenance follows the completion of initial active periodontal therapy (e.g., SRP, osseous surgery, or gingival flap surgery).

There are many treatment components involved in periodontal maintenance. The process includes the removal of plaque, calculus, and stains from tooth structures, the removal of bacterial plaque and calculus from supragingival and subgingival regions, site specific scaling and root planing, and polishing the teeth. Less treatment time should be allowed for a prophylaxis patient with a healthy mouth, and more time should be allowed for periodontal maintenance. This difference in required treatment time helps distinguish between a prophylaxis and periodontal maintenance from the patient's perspective. CDT codes are procedure based, not time based (except for select anesthesia and sedation codes).

Reimbursement

The average fee for a periodontal maintenance procedure is approximately 60% higher than the practice fee for a prophylaxis. As previously stated, the time spent and fee should differ for a prophylaxis and periodontal maintenance visit. Reimbursement varies by plan according to the criteria established in the plan document.

Downcoding

Downcoding is when a less complex procedure is reported to receive reimbursement when the actual procedure performed would not be a covered benefit. Some payors may consider this an improper billing practice. Over the years, payors have warned practices that it is improper to downcode periodontal maintenance (D4910) and report a prophylaxis (D1110) in order to receive reimbursement. In some instances, payors have demanded refunds based on specific plan document criteria.

D1110 includes the "removal of plaque, calculus and stains from the tooth structures and implants." D4910 includes the "removal of the bacterial plaque and calculus from supragingival and subgingival regions ... and polishing the teeth." However, D4910 also includes "site specific scaling and root planing, where indicated." Therefore, if scaling and root planing (SRP) is performed at the recare visit, D4910 should be reported. If only prophylaxis procedures are performed, report D1110. Always report what you do and the clinical treatment record should reflect it.

Since prophylaxis is an integral part of periodontal maintenance, it is common for practices to report D1110 in situations where D4910 may not be reimbursed. Alternating codes could be considered downcoding. It is inappropriate to downcode the periodontal maintenance procedure and report D1110 when the procedures performed at the visit meet the criteria of a periodontal maintenance procedure. Instead, report the actual procedure performed, D4910, and request the alternate benefit of a prophylaxis, D1110. The clinical notes should reflect that a prophylaxis was performed as part of the periodontal maintenance procedure to support reimbursement of the prophylaxis alternate benefit only. Occasionally, if D1110 is reported when D4910 is completed, the payor may consider this a form of unbundling and refuse to pay the claim.

Proper Reporting

Dentists are obligated to report the services that are actually provided. It is inappropriate to alternate D1110 and D4910 solely to obtain benefits for four recare visits per year. Always use the most appropriate code to describe the service actually provided regardless of benefits, or lack thereof.

When reporting periodontal maintenance, remember the prophylaxis elements are a component of the periodontal maintenance service, and the clinical record should reflect that a prophylaxis was performed as part of the maintenance procedure. Reimbursement for periodontal maintenance is highly variable and is subject to plan specific limitations.

Regardless of any plan limitations, provide the service that is clinically necessary to treat the patient's current condition or diagnosis. Do not provide or submit the service necessary to gain reimbursement. As always, be sure that the clinical records contain a clear, concise description of the procedure(s) performed and the supporting documentation necessary to justify medical necessity.

The documentation for periodontal maintenance should include the patient's current condition (such as bleeding on probing, home care, amount of

calculus, plaque, etc.) and the areas of the dentition where site specific scaling and root planing was performed. Also document that a prophylaxis was performed as part of the periodontal maintenance procedure, since this can be the basis for appeal of a denied periodontal maintenance claim due to a frequency limitation.

When periodontal maintenance is denied due to a frequency limitation, appeal the denial. Request an alternate benefit of a prophylaxis (D1110). State that a prophylaxis was performed as part of the periodontal maintenance procedure. Be sure that the clinical notes state the same. Be aware that the payor may request a copy of the clinical notes before approving the alternate benefit.

Note: If you are an in-network provider there is a significant difference between "non-billable" and "denied." Non-billable means that neither the patient nor the payor may be charged for the service. Denied means that the payor is not reimbursing for the procedure but the patient can be billed.

What About Reverting?

While periodontal disease is a chronic condition, it can be "episodic" for some patients, meaning that it can come and go over a period of time. Treatment should be based on the dentist's professional judgment to meet the patient's specific treatment needs.

If the dentist determines that the patient's current oral condition can be maintained and supported with prophylaxis treatment, then based on the clinical judgment of the dentist, a patient may return to a prophylaxis recare, with a recommended frequency (i.e., three prophylaxis visits a year). Currently there is no CDT code prophy frequency recommendation. If, in the future, active periodontal disease recurs, the patient would need to receive active periodontal therapy again (such as SRP or periodontal surgery) before returning to a periodontal maintenance recare regimen. The chronic, more advanced periodontal patient may continue periodontal maintenance therapy indefinitely unlike the patient with mild periodontal disease.

Most payors require SRP to be performed and the patient requalified for periodontal maintenance every 24 to 36 months to receive benefits for ongoing periodontal maintenance therapy. Others (e.g., many of the Delta Dental plans) provide reimbursement for D4910 recare appointments indefinitely.

Summary of D1110 vs. D4910

D1110 PROPHYLAXIS (Includes implants)	D4910 PERIODONTAL MAINTENANCE
Preventive in nature	Therapeutic in nature
Less time required	More time required
Lower fee	Higher fee
Scaling & Polishing	Scaling & Root Planing (site specific) & polishing
Less frequent probing and charting	More frequent probing and charting

The ADA's Position

In 2000, the Health Insurance Portability and Accountability Act of 1996 (HIPAA) designated Current Dental Terminology (CDT) as the standard code set to be used to report dental procedures. The ADA's Council on Dental Benefit Programs (CDBP) established the Code Maintenance Committee (CMC) to maintain CDT. Therefore, the ADA is the controlling authority on CDT and the interpretations established in its publications trump any other opinion(s) when it comes to properly reporting CDT codes.

The ADA is clear that "treatment plans must be developed according to professional standards, not according to provisions of the dental benefit contract." (*CDT 2023 Coding Companion*, Page 1) In addition, the "Golden Rules" of Procedure Coding (Page 16) include:

- "Code for what you do" is the fundamental rule to apply in all coding situations.

- After reading the full nomenclature and descriptor, select the code that matches the procedure delivered to the patient.

- If there is no applicable code, document the service using an unspecified, by report ("999") code, and include a clear and appropriate narrative.

- The existence of a procedure code does not mean that the procedure is a covered or reimbursed benefit in a dental benefit plan.

- Treatment planning is based on clinical need, not on covered services.

The following summary reviews the ADA's view on alternating D4910 and D1110 and reverting from D4910 to D1110.

Alternating

The ADA's *CDT 2023 Coding Companion: Training Guide for the Dental Team*, Page 83 states the following regarding D4910 verses D1110 recare visits following active periodontal therapy:

Periodontal Maintenance Therapy and Prophylaxis Visits

Following either surgical or non-surgical periodontal therapy the patient is placed by the treating dentist on a program of scheduled periodic periodontal maintenance (D4910) visits, which could be at various intervals (e.g., 2, 3, 4, or 6 months) depending on the patient's clinical condition. The D4910 periodontal maintenance procedure includes removal of bacterial plaque and calculus (mineralized deposits) from subgingival and supragingival tooth surfaces, site- specific scaling and root planing, and coronal tooth polishing. Between these scheduled periodontal maintenance visits the patient is also seen by the dentist for routine dental prophylaxis (tooth cleaning procedures).

May the dentist code and bill for the prophylaxis procedure (D1110 or D1120) or is this prohibited as a duplication of existing services under D4910?

Nothing in the D4910 or the D1110 (or D1120) code nomenclatures or descriptors make these procedures mutually exclusive. If the dentist determines that the patient's periodontal health can be augmented with periodic routine prophylaxis procedures (removal of plaque, calculus and stains from the tooth structures for the purpose of controlling local irritational factors), then this service should be performed and reported as D1110 or D1120, depending on the state of the dentition.

Does it make any difference if the reporting dentist for prophylaxis (D1110 or D1120) is the same dentist providing periodontal maintenance (D4910)?

No. The dentist should code and report for the services provided regardless of the provision of other services by the same or a different dentist.

Will both procedures be reimbursed by the patient's dental benefit carrier?

Reimbursement will depend upon the dental benefit plan language and the contractual policies governing covered benefits.

Thus, as the controlling authority, the ADA indicates that D4910 and D1110 can be appropriately delivered at different times for the same patient under specific circumstances.

Patient Communication

The periodontal maintenance patient often feels as if they received a prophylaxis and do not understand that periodontal maintenance is a continuation of active periodontal therapy. This can create challenges when communicating with a patient with coverage for two prophylaxis visits and two periodontal maintenance visits per benefit year. (Note: Some "Cadillac" dental plans will allow four periodontal maintenance visits plus two prophylaxis visits per benefit year.) Explain to the patient that periodontal maintenance is continuation of periodontal therapy and is treating active periodontal disease by performing site specific scaling and root planing in addition to polishing.

While explaining the need for continued periodontal maintenance is challenging, it can also be hard to explain reverting back to prophylaxis status. A good explanation could be, "While you do have periodontal disease with bone loss, your case is currently rather mild. With the periodontal treatments you have received over the past two years and your diligent homecare regimen, the doctor feels that you can return to a prophylaxis recare status. However, periodontal disease can be episodic (over the course of your lifetime), so we would like to perform a prophylaxis every four months to monitor your disease. Your dental plan allows benefits for two prophylaxis visits per year, so one of those three visits will not be reimbursed by your insurance and you will be responsible for the full fee. Congratulations, your compliance and diligence with homecare has certainly improved your overall oral health!"

Conclusion

When selecting the proper code to submit for any procedure, there are two things to remember:

1. Always report what you do – nothing more, nothing less.

2. Always appropriately document what you do in the clinical chart and on the claim form.

There is no cut and dry answer regarding the appropriateness of alternating D4910 and D1110 or reverting from D4910 to D1110. The treatment provided should be the most appropriate treatment to meet the patient's current periodontal needs. The code submitting should correlate with the actual treatment provided.

For more extensive details on this topic, refer to the ADA's *CDT 2023 Coding Companion Training Guide for the Dental Team.*

Source:

http://members.perio.org/libraries/glossary?ssopc=1

Notes

_____

_____

_____

_____

_____

_____

_____

_____

_____

_____

_____

In order to compete with the rise of corporate dentistry, many solo and smaller general dental practices are expanding their procedure mix or bringing in specialists in order to offer their patients a wider variety of services.

Documenting for Orthodontics

In order to compete with the rise of corporate dentistry, many solo and smaller general dental practices are expanding their procedure mix or bringing in specialists in order to offer their patients a wider variety of services. This allows patients to access comprehensive treatment at the same location which is very convenient and appealing to them.

Because more adult patients today are seeking a straighter smile, many general dentists have added orthodontic treatment to their procedure mix. However, the addition of orthodontic procedures in the general dentistry practice can present billing challenges for the dental team members unfamiliar with orthodontic procedures and billing.

There are various techniques and methods of orthodontic treatment today, including traditional metal brackets, clear brackets, Damon® brackets, or a series of removable appliances such as Reveal®, ClearCorrect®, etc.

However, the proper reporting for orthodontics is not based on the technique or method, but rather on the patient's dentition at the start of treatment, as well as the type of case, either limited or comprehensive.

Stages of Dentition

The stages of dentition, as defined by CDT 2023, are as follows:

Primary Dentition: Teeth developed and erupted first in order of time.

Transitional Dentition: The final phase of the transition from primary to adult teeth, in which the deciduous molars and canines are in the process of shedding and the permanent successors are emerging.

Adolescent Dentition: The dentition that is present after the normal loss of primary teeth and prior to cessation of growth that would affect orthodontic treatment.

Adult Dentition: The dentition that is present after the cessation of growth that would affect orthodontic treatment.

Limited Orthodontic Treatment

Limited orthodontic treatment includes the treatment of one arch and/or segments of both arches, closing open spaces, correcting a crossbite or uprighting a molar for a fixed partial denture, etc. Limited orthodontic treatment is appropriately reported when the treatment is limited in scope or the entire dentition is not treated. Limited orthodontic treatment does not involve the entire dentition; therefore, the fees charged are typically less than fees for a comprehensive orthodontic case.

Limited orthodontic cases are reported using one of the following CDT codes:

D8010 Limited orthodontic treatment of the primary dentition

D8020 Limited orthodontic treatment of the transitional dentition

D8030 Limited orthodontic treatment of the adolescent dentition

D8040 Limited orthodontic treatment of the adult dentition

Comprehensive Orthodontic Treatment

Comprehensive orthodontic treatment includes treatment of both arches leading to improvement of a patient's craniofacial dysfunction and/or dentofacial deformity, which may include anatomical, functional, and/or esthetic relationships. The treatment outcome should result in an improved functional, occlusal, and esthetic relationship. If the orthodontic treatment provided does not address both arches, consider reporting limited orthodontic treatment.

Comprehensive orthodontics involves a coordinated diagnosis that may include a cephalometric radiographic image with analysis, photographs, and diagnostic casts. Reveal® and other aligner techniques may not require a cephalometric radiographic image.

Comprehensive orthodontic cases are reported using one of the following CDT codes:

D8070 Comprehensive orthodontic treatment of the transitional dentition

D8080 Comprehensive orthodontic treatment of the adolescent dentition

D8090 Comprehensive orthodontic treatment of the adult dentition

Clear Aligners

While many orthodontic cases utilizing clear aligners such as Reveal® are reported for one arch as a limited case; comprehensive orthodontics may be reported for cases addressing and treating the entire dentition.

The ADA's *CDT 2023 Coding Companion Training Guide for the Dental Team* offers clarity to this frequently asked question regarding clear aligners:

"What code should be used to report treatment using clear aligners?

Coding for treatments using clear aligner therapy would be the same code that would be used for a treatment utilizing orthodontic brackets. Choice of code is dependent on the nature of the treatment (limited or comprehensive) and the stage of dental development."

Accordingly, D8090 reports an adult case when the entire dentition is addressed using clear aligners, such as Reveal®, ClearCorrect®, etc.

Post-Orthodontic Treatment Retention

Most payors consider placement of post-orthodontic retainers inclusive to the global orthodontic case fee, while others may consider retention a separate benefit. D8680 reports orthodontic retention (removal of appliances, construction and placement of retainer(s)). Retention may be fixed, removable, or a combination of the two. D8680 includes removal of active appliances and placement of retainers on one or both arches, (i.e. it is not reported per arch).

Any removable retainer adjustments after active orthodontic treatment has been completed (including placement of retention) is reported using D8681, removable orthodontic retainer adjustment. Retainer adjustments are often included in the global fee by the payors for some period after delivery. Payors may consider reimbursement if the lifetime orthodontic benefits have not been exhausted or if a new dental plan with orthodontic benefits is available. If the provider adjusting the retainer is different than the provider of the orthodontic treatment, indicate this on the claim form as this could influence the reimbursement outcome.

10

Orthodontic Benefits and Billing

Understanding orthodontic benefits is the first step in successful billing. Dental benefit plans offering orthodontic coverage or an orthodontic rider differ substantially from general dental benefits. Prior to the start of treatment, verify the patient's orthodontic benefits, if any.

Examples of questions to ask when verifying orthodontic benefits include:

- Eligibility
- Plan type (e.g., PPO, traditional, capitation, fee schedule)
- Fully insured vs. self-funded
- Age limitations
- Out-of-network benefits
- Benefit maximum
- Deductible
- Waiting period
- Percentage paid as an intial down payment
- Payment structure (e.g., monthly, quarterly, semi-annually, annually)
- If applicable, ask if the plan allows for continuation of care
- Number of active months of treatment required for reimbursement of full orthodontic benefit
- Installments paid automatically or upon claim submission
- Retention included or reimbursed separately from the case

Orthodontic benefits almost always have a lifetime maximum. Some plans offer an annual stand-alone orthodontic benefit, or share the benefit maximum with the general dental benefit maximum, so watch out for this pitfall.

Age limitation is common with orthodontic benefits (i.e., benefits applicable to patients ages 18 and under). The age limitation may also provide that the initial banding (or delivery of first set of removable appliances, clear aligners) take place prior the patient's 19th birthday.

Payment schedules vary among payors. Some payors issue monthly payments while others reimburse quarterly. A few may even make semi-annual or annual installments. These payments will either be issued automatically or 'as billed,' depending on payor specific policies. Payors that issue payments 'as billed' will not issue payment unless a claim is submitted for each periodic orthodontic visit. These periodic orthodontic visits are reported using periodic orthodontic treatment visit (D8670). Since payment methods vary among payors, a spreadsheet or tickler file should be created to track each payor. Example: Full practice fee is $5,000 ($1,000 down payment due from patient) and payor's lifetime maximum orthodontic benefit is $1,500; payor will reimburse $500 (50%) of the initial down payment and reimburse the remaining $1,000 of the lifetime benefit over the next 12-24 months. Since there are many variations among payors, it is important to be knowledgeable of each payor's criteria prior to initiating treatment.

It is also recommended that each component of orthodontic records (e.g., D0330, D0340, D0350, and D0470) be reported up front, prior to the start of treatment. This can increase cash flow for the practice and provide an early indicator of the coverage of the plan. Some payors will reimburse records in addition to the typical lifetime maximum benefits of $1,500. In other cases, the records fee is subtracted from the lifetime benefit.

Orthodontic Claim Submission

To minimize coding errors, it is important to have a clear understanding of orthodontic coding requirements. When submitting orthodontic treatment, or any treatment related to orthodontics, it is important to indicate that the treatment submitted is for orthodontic purposes. This would include orthodontic treatment, or any component of orthodontic records or other treatment performed for orthodontic purposes, such as extraction of teeth, discing between teeth, surgical access of an unerupted tooth and/or placement of a device to aid in eruption, etc.

To indicate that the procedure is related to orthodontic treatment, check "Yes" in Box 40 of the 2019 ADA Dental Claim Form. Since many dental practice management software programs default "No" in Box 40, this is a very common claim form error, especially for a general dental practice.

Submission for reimbursement or predetermination of orthodontic benefits may require additional information on the claim form. The date the appliance was placed (often referred to as the banding date) must be noted in Box 41 of the initial claim, as well as subsequent orthodontic treatment visits. The required months of treatment is indicated in Box 42. Many plans require 12 months or more of active treatment for reimbursement of full orthodontic benefits. If six months is indicated on the claim form, the payor may not render payment for the full lifetime orthodontic maximum. Failure to complete these required boxes will result in denial or payment delays.

Do not submit the actual records (i.e., photographs, diagnostic casts, etc.) unless specifically requested by the payor.

It is not unusual for a patient's plan to terminate in the middle of active orthodontic treatment and a new policy take effect. Should the new plan provide benefits for work-in-progress, a new claim will need to be submitted. Note the importance of asking whether the new plan allows for continuation of care during the insurance verification process.

To correctly submit a work-in-progress claim, the banding date (Box 41) and months in treatment (Box 42) provided on the original claim form should remain the same upon submission to the new payor. However, the procedure date listed (Box 24) will be the effective date of the new policy. The

remarks section of the claim form (Box 35) should state this claim is a "work-in-progress," as well as indicate the amount originally paid prior to the initial plan terminating. In addition, always attach or enclose all explanations of benefit (EOBs) received from the prior policy. These are common dental billing errors which unfortunately may result in the denial of work-in-progress claims.

If you are submitting a work-in-progress claim and there was no prior insurance plan or orthodontic benefits used towards the current active treatment, the work-in-progress claim is submitted essentially the same way. The difference being that any information pertaining to a prior plan payment will be omitted and replaced with a statement indicating there were no prior benefits paid for orthodontic treatment.

PPOs and Orthodontics

In addition to the PPO contract, it is imperative that the doctor read and understand the Processing Policy Manual of each contracted PPO. The Processing Policy Manual (also called a Provider Handbook) is a separate document, not part of the contract, and may be obtained by contacting the PPO provider relations department (or via the payor password-protected website). Knowledge of the processing policies of each PPO is essential regarding the specifics of orthodontic coverage.

For example, many plans with orthodontic benefits include an age limitation. However, a PPO plan may consider orthodontics provided for an adult for cosmetic purposes an optional service, thus allowing the provider to collect the full fee for the treatment from the patient. Another example of a PPO allowing orthodontic treatment as an optional service is when the treatment involves a non-traditional treatment option such as Reveal® or ClearCorrect®.

Delta Dental of Tennessee Dentist Handbook 2022 states the following regarding Orthodontics:

10

General Policy – *Orthodontics, including oral evaluations and all treatment, must be performed by a licensed dentist or his or her supervised staff, acting within the scope of applicable law. The dentist of record must perform an in-person clinical evaluation of the patient (or the telehealth equivalent where required under applicable law to be reimbursed as an alternative to an in-person clinical evaluation) to establish the need for orthodontics and have adequate diagnostic information, including appropriate radiographic imaging, to develop a proper treatment plan. Self-administered (or any type of "do it yourself") orthodontics is denied.*

There is a difference between a "denied" or "non-billable" procedure. While the payor provides no reimbursement in either case, if the claim is denied, the patient may be billed for the procedure either up to the PPO allowable amount or the fee submitted; if the claim is non-billable, the patient may not be charged.

Remember, the terms of the specific group or individual contract supersede any PPO processing policies. It is advisable to contact the payor prior to the start of treatment regarding optional services and for clarification of contract provisions.

Orthodontic benefits vary greatly, so it is important to understand the patient's plan design and any PPO provisions. This will benefit the practice when reporting orthodontic procedures and increase the likelihood of prompt payment.

Medical Necessity and Orthodontic Treatment

Orthodontic treatment is a significant investment for most families. The first question most parents ask is if their child's orthodontic treatment will be covered by their insurance.

The Affordable Care Act (ACA) requires that children under the age of 19 be offered dental benefits with the healthcare plan that includes the ten essential health benefits, one of which is orthodontics. Many parents assume this means orthodontic treatment will be covered by their medical plan. However, this is generally not the case, since routine malocclusion and jumbled teeth do not qualify. Also, a specialist may be required for treatment under ACA.

Orthodontics must be medically necessary for a medical plan to consider reimbursement. This includes the treatment of craniofacial abnormalities, severe malocclusion caused by trauma, or craniofacial disharmonies. For example, a disabled child may have severe malocclusion that impairs the patient physically and may require medically necessary orthodontic treatment.

Thorough documentation is key in proving medical necessity for orthodontic cases. When submitting this type of claim, always include documentation supporting the diagnosis for necessity of medical treatment. ⑩

Q & A

CHAPTER ELEVEN

Documentation Q & A

Q: What is a SOAP note?

A: SOAP stands for Subjective, Objective, Assessment, and Plan, as a format for recording information about dental visits. Subjective is what the patient tells you, Objective includes the clinical findings upon examination, Assessment is the diagnosis based on the subjective and objective findings, and Plan is the treatment plan and record of treatment delivered.

Q: Do I really have to document in SOAP note format?

A: No. There is no requirement for you to format your chart notes this way. It is merely a guide to help ensure you remember to document all the critical information about a procedure that you may need in the future, for both continuity of care and liability purposes. Creating a simple, repeatable format for your chart notes allows you to consistently document the important information about patient visits that you may otherwise neglect to record.

Q: Why do I need to say that the doctor ordered the radiographs? We always take the same radiographs for certain types of visits.

A: The Center for Devices and Radiological Health of the U.S. Food and Drug Administration, in collaboration with the American Dental Association, established radiology protocols based on a needs based assessment of each patient. Which radiographs are appropriate are subject to the dentist's clinical judgment on best practice regarding the approach of diagnostic imaging on an individual patient basis. The dentist must use professional judgment, a thorough clinical evaluation, consider multiple risk factors, and review the patient's health history to determine the best use of diagnostic imaging for each patient. Radiographs must be ordered by the dentist (or hygienist if state permits evaluations, diagnosis and/or treatment plans by a hygienist) based on a cursory evaluation of the patient and assessing their situation. It is inappropriate to routinely take radiographs simply because payors reimburse them at certain time intervals. Furthermore, radiographs should be of diagnostic quality and must be reviewed. Noting that the radiographs were ordered after the clinician has done a brief evaluation and that they were subsequently reviewed, with any findings noted in the chart, is an essential part of record keeping.

For more information, see the section titled "Necessity of Radiographs" within the chapter "Audits" in Practice Booster's book, *Dental Administration With Confidence.*

Q: Is it ok to use templates for quickly creating chart notes? We try to automate as much as possible to speed up the process.

A: Templates are a great starting point for chart notes, but need to be customized for the particular patient. The chart notes must accurately reflect what happened at a particular appointment with specifics about each procedure performed. If all your chart notes have the same language, you open yourself to audits. For example, if every crown that needs a buildup needs it for the same reason according to your charting, it is likely assumed that

11

the note was written in an attempt to gain reimbursement and not as an accurate reflection of the diagnosed need for treatment for that particular tooth.

Q: Does the doctor need to review and sign every entry?

A: Very commonly, chart notes are created by a member of the dental team. There is no issue with this arrangement, but the chart notes need to be reviewed for accuracy by the treating dentist. As a record that this review occurred, each note should be initialed or signed by the treating dentist. In addition, any team member(s) assisting the doctor or hygienist in treating the patient should also be listed in the chart note. If the treatment is provided by someone other than the doctor, that person should write the chart note and sign it. Remember, the chart is a legal document that the clinician is attesting as accurate. Ultimately, the dentist is responsible for the contents of the patient record. If the record has inaccurate or incomplete information, the dentist is still liable for the record as it stands. It is in the best interest of the dentist to review each and every chart note.

Q: What if something needs to be corrected in the chart?

A: Occasionally, the clinical notes need to be amended to either correct an error or to provide additional information on a later date. In these circumstances, you should make a new entry in chronological order, referring back to the date of the visit in question. Most practice management softwares lock the notes so that alterations to previous notes are not allowed. They only allow for amendments. Any amendments should include an explanation as to why the note is being changed and what changes are being made. For example, additional information that was originally left out should be marked as a "late entry", whereas inaccurate information should be marked as a "correction to previous note", both with a date

reference to the original entry. The new or corrected information should then be recorded and the new entry should be signed or initialed by the dentist.

For practices still using paper charts, it is inappropriate to alter a note in such a way as to give the appearance that the new or corrected information was part of the original note. Never erase or obliterate an entry in a patient chart. According to Dental Records (American Dental Association, 2010), Wite-Out® and markers should never be used to correct an entry. Although most states allow providers to denote corrections with a thin line, the original wrong entry must remain readable and any additions or corrections must be dated and initialed. The ADA also warns dentists not to leave blank lines between entries with the intent to add something at a later date, because that could be construed as an alteration. Also, inserting words or phrases in an entry could be interpreted as an alteration. If you need to record additional information at a later date, the ADA instructs dentists to make a new entry in chronological order, referring back to the date of the visit in question. Do not run the risk of making a potential problem worse by altering the patient record after the fact. Verify state laws for legally defined appropriate methods for correcting or amending a clinical record, or contact your malpractice carrier for recommendations.

Q: What is the 21st Century Cures Act and how is it affecting treatment documentation?

A: The 21st Century Cures Act is a federal law passed in 2016 to streamline the exchange of health information and increase the speed in which advances in healthcare are brought to the public. Further revisions to the Act in 2020 focused on preventing information blocking with electronic health records. Two main parts of this revision included provisions for interoperability (allowing the exchange of patient records and information seamlessly between different softwares) and

Open Notes, which mandates providing patients unrestrained access to their electronic health information in a format that is "easy to understand, secure, and updated automatically." In practice, this means patients have to have immediate access to patient records when they ask for it, including all chart notes and financial records. Likely, practice management softwares will include patient portals, where patients can access these records on demand through the internet. This unrestrained access will mean more "eyes on the chart" than ever before, and thus more scrutiny than ever before. Now more than ever, providers need to be cautious about what information they put in their documentation. It is in the best interest of clinicians to keep their clinical charting clinical and not personal. Avoid comments that could be construed as negative about a patient's behavior or statements that may open the practice to litigation or censure.

Q: What about narratives? Can I repeatedly use the narratives I know will most likely result in reimbursement?

A: Narratives have long been a way to provide dental insurance payors with information they need that supports the procedures reported. These are often written in the "Remarks" section of the ADA claim form. Narratives should be short, legible, factual, and relevant as to why the procedure was necessary. They should clearly support the need for treatment based on information found in the clinical record. If the narrative does not match the information in the clinical record, including images, periodontal charts, and written notes, it may be seen as an attempt to misrepresent the procedure. Stock or canned narratives that are repeated frequently for similar procedures may also be seen as an attempt to gain reimbursement instead of proper documentation, therefore the narrative should be created jointly with the clinical team.

Narratives should be limited to 80 characters, including spaces and punctuation. Practice management softwares may allow for additional text, but that text may be clipped or truncated when passing through the insurance clearinghouse, meaning the full message may not be received by the payor. Longer narratives or messages should be processed as a separate attachment to the submission. More and more frequently, payors are asking for copies of the actual chart notes from the date of service (and any amendments) instead of a separate narrative. This again opens the clinical notes to scrutiny and presents an opportunity for the payor to raise questions. This is a further reason for clinical notes to be accurate and thorough.

Glossary

Glossary

A

Abscess – Localized inflammation that can be acute or chronic, typically includes the collection of pus and swelling. Generally associated with tissue destruction and most often secondary to infection.

Abutment – An abutment is a connecting element that supports a prosthesis (e.g., an abutment supported prosthesis).

Adjudication – The automated processing of a claim with or without review.

Adjunct/Adjunctive – Additional treatment performed, secondary to the primary treatment.

Affordable Care Act (ACA) – A combination of two separate pieces of legislation – the Patient Protection and Affordable Care Act (P.L. 111-148) and the Health Care and Education Reconciliation Act of 2010 (P.L. 111-152) – that, together expand Medicaid coverage to millions of low-income Americans and makes numerous improvements to both Medicaid and the Children's Health Insurance Program (CHIP).

ALARA – Acronym for "As Low As Reasonably Achievable." ALARA is a radiation safety principle for minimizing radiation doses and releases of radioactive materials by employing all reasonable methods. ALARA is not only a sound safety principle, but is a regulatory requirement defined by Title 10, Section 20.1003 of the Code of Federal Regulations for all radiation safety programs.

Allowable Charge – The maximum amount of benefit allowed for a dental procedure per the indemnity or the PPO plan contract.

Alternate Benefit – A provision of a dental plan allowing the payor to provide a less expensive benefit or a lower reimbursement for a non-covered procedure. For example, the payor reimburses for an amalgam restoration when the doctor actually performed a composite restoration on a molar.

Anesthesia – Elimination of sensation; pain.

Ankylosis – A rare condition in which the tooth is fused to the surrounding alveolar bone in an area of previous partial root resorption.

Anterior – A reference to the teeth and tissues found in the front of the mouth - mandibular and maxillary central incisors, lateral incisors, and canines (cuspids) are considered to be anterior teeth. The description of permanent anterior teeth in the Universal/National Tooth Numbering System includes teeth 6 through 11 (maxillary), and 22 through 27 (mandibular); anterior primary teeth in the Universal/National Tooth Numbering System are titled C through H (maxillary), and M through R (mandibular). Anterior may also refer to the front region/area of the oral cavity.

Apnea – Temporary cessation of breathing, especially during sleep.

Arthralgia – Pain associated with a joint.

Assignment of Benefits – Authorization by the patient for dental plan benefits to be paid directly to the provider of the service (i.e., the doctor).

Atrophy – A wasting away of tissue, muscle or bone due to injury or disease.

Audit – A review of records by a payor to ensure providers are upholding responsibilities regarding plan(s) specifications, along with applicable federal and state laws. Any violation found during an audit could result in the payor's request for repayment of funds paid to the doctor, sanctions, being dropped as a contracted provider, or referral to a State Dental Board for further review.

Auto Adjudication – The automated processing of a claim without human review.

Autogenous Graft – A soft tissue graft that uses tissue taken from the patient. See "non-autogenous graft."

Avulsion – Separation of a tooth from its socket, usually due to trauma.

B

Balance Billing – A request for the patient to pay the difference between the amount the practice charges and the amount the insurance paid.

Barrier Membrane – A thin material used in regenerative procedures. Commonly placed over a fresh bone graft and can be resorbable or non-resorbable. Also known as Guided Tissue Regeneration (GTR).

Basic Services – A category of services referring to covered oral procedures. These services usually consist of routine restorations, such as composite and amalgam restorations. This varies by dental plan.

Benign – Non-malignant neoplasm; non-life threatening.

Bilateral – Both sides of an arch in the mouth.

Biopsy – The removal of a piece of tissue for a histologic evaluation. This does not describe the microscopic evaluation performed by the pathologist or pathology laboratory.

Bonding – A technique in which 2 or more components are attached or affixed by chemical and/or mechanical adhesion.

Bruxism – Clenching and grinding of teeth.

Buccal – Relating to the cheek or the surface of a posterior tooth next to the cheek.

Bursitis – A painful inflammation of the bursa.

Business Associates (BA) – Anyone who provides services for the covered entity and has access to the covered entity's patient information (e.g., an IT company).

By Report – A brief narrative describing the dental procedure performed; required when reporting the CDT codes that have the words "by report" in the nomenclature.

C

Calculus – A hard residue on the teeth formed through mineralization of dead bacteria in dental plaque which adheres to teeth and prosthetic appliances; also known as tartar.

Caldwell Luc Procedure – A surgical procedure named for American surgeon, George Caldwell and French laryngologist, Henri Luc. The procedure involves an incision through the mouth into the maxillary sinus. This is often performed to clear blocked or infected sinus cavities or to remove tooth fragments.

Cancer – A group of diseases caused by the growth of abnormal cells.

Cantilever Extension – The portion of a fixed prosthesis extending past the abutment to which it is attached, having no support on the other side.

CARES Act – Signed into law on March 27, 2020, this over $2 trillion relief package provided fast and direct economic assistance for American workers, families, and small businesses, and preserved jobs for American industries.

Caries – Frequently used term for tooth decay.

Carrier (Payor) – A third-party company who administers insurance plan benefits.

Cementoenamel Junction (CEJ) – Junction of the enamel of the crown and the cementum of the root of a tooth.

Center for Disease Control (CDC) – The U.S. federal health protection agency, working 24/7 to protect America from health and safety threats, both foreign and domestic. Its main goal is to protect public health and safety through the control and prevention of disease, injury, and disability in the U.S. to increase the health security of our nation.

Centers for Medicare and Medicaid Services (CMS) – The federal agency (part of the U.S. Department of Health and Human Services) responsible for the administration of Medicare, Medicaid, Children's Health Insurance Program (CHIP), HIPAA, and the Clinical Laboratory Improvement Amendments (CLIA) programs. CMS also maintains the Healthcare Common Procedure Coding System (HCPCS) code set and ICD-10-CM code set.

Chart – The chart contains, but is not limited to, documentation regarding treatment recommended and/or provided and the necessity of that treatment, dates and the purpose of each visit, radiographic images, photographs, medication prescriptions, diagnosis, laboratory prescriptions, reports of the results of consultations with other healthcare providers, and referral information. A chart also contains documentation of all communication with the patient, whether by phone, fax, text, email, Skype, etc. A chart can be in electronic or paper form and is a part of the overall patient record.

Claim – A written request for benefit payment from an insurance carrier/payor. A claim form may be submitted to the payor by the patient or the provider.

Claim Form – The paper form or electronic format used to submit a request for benefit payment. These forms are specific as to dental and medical claims. The current and appropriate form must be submitted.

Cleft Lip – Congenital abnormality occurring when the tissue of the lip fails to form properly during pregnancy. This results in a split (i.e., cleft) in the lip creating an opening between the mouth and the nose. This cleft may be unilateral, bilateral, median, or complete. A cleft lip typically only affects the upper lip and is often associated with a cleft palate.

Cleft Palate – Congenital deformity resulting in lack of fusion of the soft and/or hard palate, either partial or complete.

Clinical – Direct patient care (i.e., the diagnosis and treatment of the patient).

Clinical Attachment Loss (CAL) – Involves the loss of alveolar bone support and gingival attachment as the periodontal fibers migrate apically from the cementoenamel junction (CEJ) due to periodontal toxins in plaque.

Clinical Crown – The portion of the tooth above the gum line.

Clinical Laboratory Improvement Amendments of 1988 (CLIA) – U.S. federal regulatory standards that apply to all clinical laboratory testing on human specimens, except clinical trial and basic research.

Closed Fracture (Bone) – An injury in which a bone is fractured (i.e., broken) but does not break through the skin.

Closed Fracture (Tooth) – An injury in which a tooth is chipped or fractured (i.e., broken) but the pulp is not exposed.

Cone Beam Computed Tomography Imaging Technology (CBCT) – A 2D or 3D radiographic image.

Congenital – Condition that exist at birth.

Connective Tissue (CT) Grafts – Donor tissue is taken from the patient and is placed in the area of gingival recession to obtain root coverage.

Contract – An agreement between a provider (doctor) and an insurance payor, usually pertaining to the doctor agreeing to participate as an in-network provider for the dental plan.

Contract Dentist – A doctor who has signed a contract (e.g., with a PPO, Delta Dental Premier, Cigna Dental Network Savings Program, etc.) agreeing to participate in an insurance plan by providing services under specific terms and conditions as stated in the contract.

Coping – A thin covering of the coronal portion of a tooth, usually devoid of anatomic contour, that can be used as a definitive restoration.

Core Buildup – Refers to building up of coronal structure when there is insufficient retention for a separate extracoronal restoration. A core buildup is not a filler to eliminate any undercut, box form, or concave irregularity in a preparation.

Corporate Integrity Agreement – The Office of the Inspector General (OIG) negotiates corporate integrity agreements (CIAs) with healthcare providers and other entities as part of the settlement of federal healthcare program investigations arising under a variety of civil false claims statutes. Providers or entities agree to the obligations, and in exchange, OIG agrees not to seek their exclusion from participation in Medicare, Medicaid, or other federal healthcare programs.

Coverage – The benefits available for dental procedures as outlined in the dental plan's summary plan description (usually 15-to-20 page patient booklet) and the plan document (usually 100 to 200 pages) as administered by the payor.

Covered Entity (CE) – Any business working in the healthcare industry that provides treatment and electronically transmits any health information in connection with transactions for which the Department of Health and Human Services (HHS) has adopted standards.

Covered Services – Dental or medical procedures for which the plan provides reimbursement.

COVID-19 – Illness caused by a coronavirus called SARS-CoV-2, primarily spread from person to person. Older adults and people who have severe underlying medical conditions like heart or lung disease or diabetes seem to be at higher risk for developing more serious complications from COVID-19 illness.

Craniofacial – Relating to the face and cranium.

Current Dental Terminology (CDT) – A code set defined by the American Dental Association (ADA) that doctors are required to follow when reporting dental procedures to an insurance company for reimbursement and on patient billing statements.

Current Procedural Terminology (CPT) – A code set defined by the American Medical Association (AMA) that medical and dental providers are required to follow when reporting medical procedures (on a medical claim form) to an insurance company for reimbursement and on patient billing statements.

Cyst – An abnormal growth, which can occur in any part of the body. Cysts are characterized by a closed sac-like structure, consisting of a membrane lining, and filled with fluid, air, tissue, pus, or other materials.

D

Debridement – The gross removal of supra and subgingival calculus.

Dental Benefits Consultant – A licensed doctor who reviews dental claims for medical necessity and makes a recommendation regarding payment to the insurance payor based upon benefit guidelines per the dental plan document. For further information regarding dental benefits consultants, visit www.aadc.org.

Dental Implant – The artificial replacement of a tooth root.

Descriptor – Text used to further define a CDT code and its intended use.

Diabetes – A group of metabolic diseases characterized by a chronic elevation in blood sugar (i.e., hyperglycemia). Uncontrolled diabetes creates an increased risk of periodontal disease along many other serious health issues.

Diastema – A space between two adjacent teeth, usually a large space between anterior teeth.

Digital Imaging and Communication in Medicine (DICOM) – The set of international standards followed when sharing digital images with other providers

Discing Teeth – An orthodontic related procedure that uses a disc to remove a small amount of interproximal enamel to create adequate space for the eruption or movement of other teeth. Discing may also be utilized to create space when aligning crowded permanent teeth, typically anterior.

Distal – Surface of a tooth farthest from the midline of the dental arch.

Durable Medical Equipment (DME) – Any equipment providing therapeutic benefits for a patient's need as a result of illness or certain medical conditions.

E

ECC – Early Childhood Caries.

Edentulous – Describes a maxillary or mandibular arch without teeth.

EHR – Electronic Health Record. A digital version of the patient's paper chart.

Employee Retirement Income Security Act (ERISA) – The Employee Retirement Income Security Act of 1974 (ERISA) is a federal law that sets minimum standards for most voluntarily established pension and health plans in private industry to provide protection for individuals in these plans

Encounter – Contact between a patient and a healthcare provider who is responsible for diagnosis and treatment.

Epulis – A gingival growth, typically benign.

Explanation of Benefits (EOB) – Document received from the insurance payor when processing of a claim has been completed. The EOB explains the benefit paid and how the benefit was determined. If an EOB is from a PPO, it also explains the patient's financial responsibility.

Exposed Roots – The crown of the tooth is missing, and the exposed root is at or above the gum line.

F

Facial – The surface of a tooth directed toward the lips or cheeks (i.e., the buccal and labial surfaces) and opposite the lingual surface.

Fistula – An abnormal opening between two organs of the body. Fistulas may be congenital or the result of disease, injury, or surgery.

G

Fixed Partial Denture (FPD) – (Also known as a bridge.) Usually consists of two retainer crowns and a pontic to replace a missing tooth. A bridge can be longer and involve more retainer crowns and/or pontics. A fixed partial denture (FPD) is permanently affixed to the retainer crown teeth with dental cement or by bonding.

Flipper – (Also referred to as a Stayplate.) A removable partial denture typically placed for a short period of time and may or may not have clasps. Sometimes referred to as an interim partial; so named because it can be easily flipped out of place with the tongue.

Focused Review – A period of time set by the payor requiring manual review of all claims for a select group of dental procedure codes submitted by a particular provider to ensure all treatments have the appropriate supporting documentation. During this period of time, the provider may be required to submit narratives, radiographs, photographs, chart notes, and other documentation to support the treatment submitted for reimbursement to ensure plan contract guidelines are being met.

Foreign Body – Any object found in the body that is not naturally occurring and does not belong there. A foreign body may be the result of an accident, such as a splinter lodged in soft tissue, or an object placed in a natural orifice (e.g., a child who swallows a coin or places small objects in an ear or nose).

Fracture – A crack or break of bone, cartilage, or teeth. A fracture may be either open or closed. See "closed fracture" and "open fracture."

Fraud – Occurs when an individual receives benefits paid by an insurance plan due to the filing of a false claim, inflated claim, or the billing of services not actually performed. Fraud is determined by a court of law.

Frenectomy – Frena are small folds of tissue located in the mouth. A frenectomy is a simple surgical procedure to loosen or release these bands, often performed by an oral and maxillofacial surgeon to increase the range of motion of the tongue (removing the lingual frenum) or to close a gap in a patient's upper front teeth (removing the labial frenum).

Frenuloplasty – A procedure which alters or repairs the frenum without completely removing it.

Frenum/frenulum – Interchangeable terms for a fold of skin or mucous membrane which restricts movement of a body part or organ (e.g., the small band of tissue that connects the underside of the tongue to the floor of the mouth).

Furcation – The area of a multi rooted tooth where the roots meet or connect with one another

G

Genetic Analysis – Methods for studying the hereditary characteristics of organisms.

Gingivectomy – The removal of gingiva (soft tissue) from around a tooth.

Gingivoplasty – A surgical procedure that reshapes the gingiva (soft tissue) around a tooth.

GP – General practitioner (or general dentist).

Guided Tissue Regeneration (GTR) – (Also referred to as a barrier membrane procedure.) A membrane is placed under the gingival tissue and over the bone to prevent epithelial cells from inhibiting the regeneration of new bone. The barrier membrane may hold a bone graft in place. Barrier membranes may be resorbable or nonresorbable.

H

HCPCS – Healthcare Common Procedure Coding System.

Health and Human Services (HHS) – The United States Department of Health & Human Services, also known as the Health Department, is a cabinet-level executive branch department of the U.S. federal government with the goal of protecting the health of all Americans and providing essential human services.

HIPAA – Health Insurance Portability and Accountability Act of 1996.

HITECH – Health Information Technology for Economic and Clinical Health.

Hugger Bridge – Consists of two resin retainer "wings" and one pontic (a type of Maryland bridge). Usually the "wings" on a hugger bridge attach to both the facial and lingual of the retainer teeth. It is composed of tooth colored hybrid composite material.

I

Iatrogenic – Trauma or condition caused by the treating doctor.

Ilium – The broad, flaring portion of the hip bone.

Incisal – The cutting or biting edges of the cuspid and incisor teeth.

Incision and Drainage (I & D) – A procedure that involves an incision made to drain an area of infection

Indirect Restoration – A restoration fabricated outside of the mouth (e.g., a crown or onlay).

Informed Consent – Consent from the patient to proceed with treatment after being presented with all necessary information to make an informed decision regarding such treatment.

Interim – A provisional prosthesis designed for use over a limited period of time, after which it is replaced by a more definitive restoration. Typically refers to a denture or other appliance used during the healing phase of treatment, or to prepare for further treatment.

Interim Therapeutic Restoration (ITR) – Placement of an adhesive restorative material following caries debridement by hand or other method. Performed to aid in the management of early childhood caries.

Intermediate Restorative Material (IRM) – A medicative material typically used after removing extensive decay that remains in the tooth until the patient returns for definitive treatment.

L

LDA/LDAA – Local Delivery of Antimicrobial Agents such as Atridox®, Arestin®, PerioChip®, etc.

Lesion – Wound, injury, or pathological change in tissues.

Lingual – The area around the tongue or the surface of the tooth located near the tongue; opposite of facial or buccal.

Locum Tenens – A doctor who is filling in for another doctor who is away from the practice for a limited period of time (i.e., regular doctor is ill or is on vacation). A locum tenens doctor fills in to take care of patient emergencies, perform hygiene evaluations, or complete treatment.

Long Face Syndrome – A malocclusion characterized by a long, narrow face; steep mandibular plane angle; and Class II Division 1 dental/skeletal relationship with anterior crowding and associated oral cavity breathing.

M

Magnetic Resonance Imaging (MRI) – A scanning technique used to diagnose and evaluate soft tissue.

Malignant – A neoplasm having the properties of localized dysplasia and metastasis; destructive growth.

Major Services – These services, as determined by the payors, usually consist of crowns, fixed partial dentures, removable prosthetics, implant services, and endodontic therapy.

Mandible – The lower jaw.

Mandibular – Pertaining or referring to the mandible.

Maryland Bridge – A resin bonded bridge fabricated to replace a missing tooth that consists of 2 retainer wings bonded to the lingual or facial of the teeth adjacent to the missing tooth and attached to the pontic replacing the missing tooth. Maryland bridges are usually made of porcelain fused to metal, resin, or a porcelain/ceramic material. This bridge is named for the University of Maryland, where it was developed.

Maxilla – The upper jaw.

Maxillary – Pertaining or referring to the maxilla.

Mesial – The surface of the tooth closest to the center or middle line of the dental arch.

Mineral Trioxide Aggregate (MTA) – A filling material used to create a plug for the apex of a tooth to repair a perforated root, to treat apexogenesis, or may be used to treat internal root resorption.

Multi-Slice Computer Tomography (MSCT) – A scan that captures an image of a specific part of the body.

N

Narrative – A brief written report describing the dental procedure performed with the goal of proving medical or dental necessity.

National Association of Dental Plans (NADP) – The representative and recognized resource of the dental benefits industry. NADP is the largest non-profit, national trade association focused exclusively on the entire dental benefits industry (i.e., dental HMOs, dental PPOs, discount dental plans and dental indemnity products). National Association of Insurance Commissioners (NAIC) – The U.S. standard-setting and regulatory support organization created and governed by the chief insurance regulators from the 50 states, the District of Columbia and five U.S. territories. Through the NAIC state insurance regulators establish standards and best practices, conduct peer review, and coordinate regulatory oversight.

National Practitioner Data Bank (NPDB) – An electronic database created by Congress to maintain information regarding malpractice payments and other adverse actions pertaining to healthcare providers, entities, and suppliers. Federal law mandates what type of actions may be reported, who may report these actions, and who may obtain the reports. This confidential information is obtained and reviewed only by authorized organizations to determine licensing, credentialing, privileging, and employment decisions.

NEC – Not elsewhere classified.

Neoplasm – Abnormal tissues that can be benign or malignant.

Nomenclature – Written definition of a procedure code.

Non-Autogenous Graft – A soft tissue graft that uses tissue not obtained from the patient. See "autogenous graft."

Notice of Privacy Practices – A written document provided to patients outlining the practice's policies regarding the use and disclosure of protected health information (PHI). This documentation is required under HIPAA.

O

Obstructive Sleep Apnea – Condition that occurs when soft tissues of the throat collapse during sleep, resulting in restriction of the airway, snoring, absence of breathing (apnea), and a decrease in oxygen in the bloodstream. Occlusal – The chewing surfaces of the molar and premolar teeth.

Occlusal Guard – A removable appliance placed to protect against tooth structure loss in patients who brux, clench, and/or grind their teeth.

Occupational Safety and Health Administration (OSHA) – A department of the federal government that enforces a set of federal laws and regulations to ensure the safety and health of employees in the workplace.

Office of Civil Rights (OCR) – The U.S. Department of Health and Human Services (HHS) Office for Civil Rights (OCR), enforces federal civil rights laws, conscience and religious freedom laws, the Health Insurance Portability and Accountability Act (HIPAA) Privacy, Security, and Breach Notification Rules, and the Patient Safety Act and Rule, which together protect your fundamental rights of nondiscrimination, conscience, religious freedom, and health information privacy at covered entities.

Office of Inspector General (OIG) – The Office of Inspector General assists the Department of Health and Human Services (HHS) detect and prevent waste, abuse, and fraud and also helps improve the efficiency of HHS programs. Most of the OIG resources and responsibilities lie in overseeing HHS, but they also extend to Centers for Disease Control and Prevention (CDC), National Institutes of Health (NIH), and the Food and Drug Administration (FDA).

Orthotic – Describes a device used to support and immobilize muscles and joints, thus restoring and improving function of the body part. An orthotic device is commonly used to treat TMD/TMJ.

P

Palliative Treatment – Alleviating pain or discomfort, without dealing with the underlying cause of the problem or condition.

Pathology – The science of the causes and effects of disease. Also refers to the branch of medicine specializing in laboratory specimens of body tissue for diagnostic purposes.

Payor (Carrier) – A third-party company who administers insurance plan benefits.

Peer Review Organization (PRO) – An organization established by an amendment of the Tax Equity and Fiscal Responsibility Act of 1982 (TEFRA) to provide review of medical services delivered primarily in a hospital setting and/or in conjunction with care provided under both Medicare and Medicaid programs. In addition to reviewing and monitoring services, PROs can also invoke sanctions, penalties, or other corrective actions for noncompliance in organization standards.

Periodontal – The supporting soft tissues and bony structures that surround the teeth.

Personal Protective Equipment (PPE) – includes protective clothing, gowns, gloves, face shields, goggles, face masks, and respirators or other equipment designed to protect the wearer from injury or the spread of infection or illness.

Plan Document – Document outlining the details of the plan, including exclusions, limitations, etc. This document can be up to 200 pages and may only be obtained by the employee from the Human Resources Department, if it is an employer sponsored group plan or from the insurance company, if an individual policy.

Platelet Rich Plasma (PRP) – The process of spinning the patient's blood and obtaining a concentrated source of autologous platelets. The platelets are rich in growth factors that stimulate bone growth in combination with a bone graft.

Point of Service – A point of service (POS) plan is a type of managed care plan that is a hybrid of HMO and PPO plans. Like an HMO, participants designate in-network physicians or dentists as their primary care providers. But, like a PPO, patients may go outside of the provider network for healthcare services. See www.healthcoverageguide.org for more information.

Porcelain Fused to Metal (PFM) – The method used to fabricate a crown or bridge, whereby tooth colored porcelain covering is fused to metal to make the crown look more like a natural tooth.

Preventive Resin Restoration (PRR) – Restores an active carious lesion in the occlusal enamel of a permanent tooth with moderate or high caries risk that does not extend into the dentin. Preparation of the tooth must be performed by the doctor. This procedure includes placement of a sealant in radiating noncarious pits or fissures.

Privacy Contact – The individual within the practice designated to be responsible for providing information, receiving complaints, and administering patients' rights, as stated in the practice's Notice of Privacy Practices. This employee appointed position is required under HIPAA.

Privacy Officer – The individual within the practice designated to be responsible for the development and implementation of the policies and procedures that are necessary in order to maintain compliance under HIPAA. This includes proper training of all team members and necessary documentation. This position is required under HIPAA.

Privacy Rule – Standard that protects patient records and any other information related to the patient's health. This rule must be followed by all dental practices as a dental practice is considered to be a covered entity under HIPAA.

Processing Policy Manual – Policies, restrictions, and rules outlined by payors in a manual which contracted providers must follow in addition to the contract.

Prosthesis – An artificial body part. In dentistry, this could be dentures or an artificial temporomandibular joint. Protected Health Information (PHI) – Information regarding a patient's health care is considered protected information under HIPAA. This includes, but is not limited to, clinical and financial information regarding the patient's health care and patient demographics.

Pulp – Blood vessels, connective tissue, and nerve tissue inside the pulp chamber of a tooth.

Q

Quadrant – One half of a dental arch. Each quadrant begins at the midline of the lower or upper arch and extends outward to the last tooth and is one of four equal sections of the mouth.

R

Rebase – The refitting of a denture achieved by replacement of the base material (the pink portion).

Records – The patient record may include, but is not limited to, the following: treatment plans, financial transactions, radiographic images, photographic images, study models, and the patient's clinical notes and chart.

Reline – The process of resurfacing the tissue side of a denture with new base material.

Reimbursement – Payment made by the payor to the subscriber (insured) or the provider for services received by an eligible patient.

Remapping (Downcoding) – A practice by payors whereby the least expensive alternative treatment (LEAT) benefit is provided.

Resection – Removal of all or part of a damaged or diseased organ or structure of the body.

Residual Tooth Roots – Remaining root(s) below the gum line after the loss of the crown of a natural tooth. Rider – An amendment within a group dental plan that can add or delete benefits and/or limitations of the plan (e.g., implant or periodontal rider).

Root Canal Therapy (RCT) – (Also referred to as endodontic therapy.) Treatment which consists of removing the damaged or diseased pulp from the root of the tooth and obturating the roots, thus the canals are filled with a material, such as gutta-percha, and sealed.

S

Scaling and Root Planing (SRP) – An active procedure to treat periodontal disease. The removal of plaque, calculus, and toxins surrounding the teeth and the root surfaces where pocketing has occurred due to the loss of bone.

Security Rule (HIPAA) – Standard set of rules to be followed by covered entities (CEs) and business associates (BAs) that protect and ensure the security, confidentiality, and integrity of electronic information containing protected health information (PHI).

Sequela – A complication or condition that arises as a direct result of an injury.

Sinus – A cavity or hollow area within bone or other tissue. This may occur in any part of the body, but typically the term is used to describe the cavities in the facial bones connecting with the nasal cavities.

Snap-on-Smile – A custom made set of teeth that fits over the existing teeth of the arch. The set is made of a thin material and looks like natural teeth. In addition to using this appliance as a cosmetic appliance, it can also be used to stabilize mobile teeth, as an interim partial denture, or as a retainer after the completion of active orthodontic treatment to maintain arch form. It may also be used as a space maintainer until a fixed partial denture or an implant and crown can be placed.

Stainless Steel Crown (SSC) – A type of crown fabricated using nickel chrome. Commonly used as a restoration for primary teeth with a large amount of decay lacking sufficient tooth structure for a filling restoration. However, a SSC can also be used for a permanent tooth restoration in some situations.

Stayplate – See "Flipper."

Summary Plan Description – A summary booklet (usually 15-to-20 pages) provided by law to participants outlining the benefits of the Plan Document.

Surgical Stent – A custom-made clear mold of the arch that is modified for use as a guide for the doctor to adjust bone following full mouth extractions. A surgical stent may also be used to achieve close approximation of tissues.

T

Third-Party Administrator (TPA) – The third-party administrator is responsible for the collection of payment from the employer, determination of benefits, and processing of benefit payments for claims. For insured plans, the third-party assumes financial risks and for self-funded (ERISA) plans the third-party only performs administrative services on behalf of the self-funded plan. The third-party may also provide a PPO provider network.

TMJ Dysfunction – A disorder of the TMJ (temporomandibular joint) and muscles of mastication resulting in clicking joints, pain, restricted movement of the mandible, and other symptoms.

TMJ/TMD – TMJ is an acronym for temporomandibular joint. TMD is an acronym for temporomandibular dysfunction. Each term refers to a group of symptoms, including pain, affecting the temporomandibular joint.

Tooth Bounded Space – A space resulting from one or more missing teeth with a remaining tooth on either side of the space.

Torus/Tori – A bulging projection of bone on the mandible or maxilla.

Treacher-Collins Syndrome – A rare genetic disorder characterized by multiple abnormalities in the development of the face and head.

Trismus – A spasm of the jaw muscles characterized by the inability to open the mouth or jaw.

U

Unbundling – The separation of a dental procedure into discrete components, charging separately for each component, resulting in a higher total fee.

Unilateral – One side of an arch in the mouth.

Upcoding – Fraudulent practice of reporting an inaccurate code of increased complexity to increase reimbursement. U.S. Department of Health & Human Services (HHS) – Designed to enhance and protect the health and wellbeing of all Americans by providing for effective health and human services and fostering advances in medicine, public health, and social services.

Usual, Customary, and Reasonable (UCR) – Average fees charged by a doctor in a specific region or ZIP code for procedures. UCR is calculated by payors using data obtained from fees submitted on claim forms by doctors from specific regions. Most commonly the ZIP code determines the allowable fee.

Utilization Review – A review by the payor of frequent procedures reported by a provider. This review is sometimes used to audit the provider to ensure accurate reporting of procedures and to detect overutilization or overbilling.

W

Waiting Period – A time period starting on the effective date of coverage as stated within the patient's plan document, which must be satisfied prior to receiving benefit. This waiting period is usually a period of six to twelve months for basic or major classification of services.

Workers' Comp – Workers' compensation provides medical expenses, lost wages, and rehabilitation costs to employees who are injured or become ill "in the course and scope" of their job. It also pays death benefits to families of employees who are killed on the job.

Z

Z-plasty – A surgical technique in which a Z shaped incision is made. This type of incision is often used for scar revisions.

Notes

Index

Index

Notes

Acknowledgments

Thank you to the following for this current 2023 edition:
Micheline Paige (design/layout), Tiffany Wesley (production/editing/design), Tija Hunter (contributor/editing), Dr. Greg Grobmyer (contributor/editing), Leslie Icenogle (contributor/editing), Jessica Feigl (editing), Lindsay Salazar (editing), Mason Blair (editing), Jim DiMarino (editing), Jonni Anderson (editing), Amara Cashion (editor). Also, thank you to the entire Practice Booster team for their dedication and hard work.

About the author

Dr. Blair is President of Dr. Charles Blair & Associates, Inc. He has authored/coauthored 15 books and countless articles. His latest publications include: *Dental Coding With Confidence: The "Go To" Dental Coding Guide; Dental Administration With Confidence: The "Go To" Guide for Insurance Administration; Medical Dental Cross Coding With Confidence: The Definitive Guide to Cross Coding; Dental Documentation With Confidence: The "Go To" Documentation Guide for the Clinical Team, Dental Technology With Confidence: The Insurance Guide to Innovative Procedures, and Practice Booster's Insurance Solutions Newsletter.*

PracticeBooster.com is his breakthrough online dental system to recover lost revenue and eliminate costly dental coding errors.

A graduate of Erskine College, Dr. Blair earned his Doctor of Dental Surgery at the University of North Carolina at Chapel Hill.Dr. Blair holds degrees in Accounting, Business Administration, Mathematics, and Dental Surgery. He is a highly regarded speaker for national, state, and local dental groups, study clubs, and other organizations. His leading edge presentations on coding, profitability, and the business side of dentistry are well-regarded nationwide. Additionally, he has assisted thousands of practices across the country in maximizing their profits through his proven *Revenue Enhancement Program.*

For more information on our full range of services, products, publications, and speaking availability call 704.829.3194 or visit www.practicebooster.com/store.

Products and Publications:

- **PracticeBooster.com** (Online Dental Coding/Resource System and Insurance Solutions Newsletter)

- **Dental Coding With Confidence:** The "Go To" Dental Coding Guide

- **Dental Administration With Confidence:** The "Go To" Guide For Insurance Administration

- **Medical Dental Cross Coding With Confidence**: The Definitive Guide to Cross Coding

- **Dental Documentation With Confidence:** The "Go To" Documentation Guide for the Clinical Team

- **Dental Technology With Confidence:** The Insurance Guide to Innovative Procedures

Speaking and Consulting:

- **Revenue Enhancement Program**

- **Coordination of Benefits Training 1:1**

- **Speaker Availability**

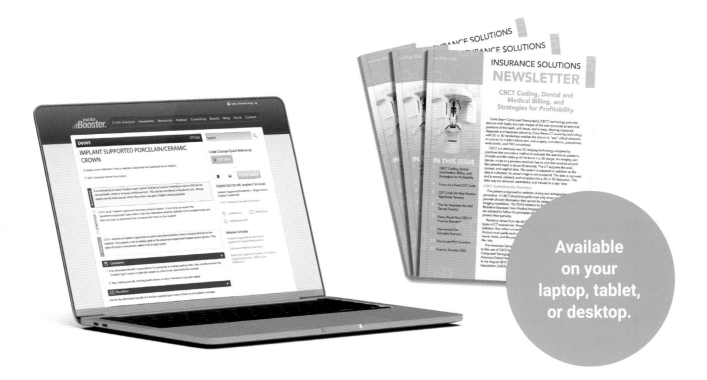

Available on your laptop, tablet, or desktop.

Practice Booster

Understanding how to properly report dental procedures and provide the proper documentation required by payors is essential to receiving timely payment for dental services. We're here to help!

Your annual subscription to Practice Booster includes:

· Exclusive access to Code Advisor, a powerful online database of CDT codes, featuring an in-depth review of proper CDT coding, billing tips, and more

· Access to online resource center featuring Q&As, sample forms and checklists, and much more

· Email/phone support available for your dental and medical coding questions

· A subscription to **Insurance Solutions Newsletter**

· Insurance Solutions Newsletter covers an array of topics, including proper insurance coding and administration, practice administration, and much more.

· Six print issues (every other month)

· Exclusive access to online archives of the past 3 years' issues

· Email/phone support available for your dental and medical coding questions

Order form on page 116

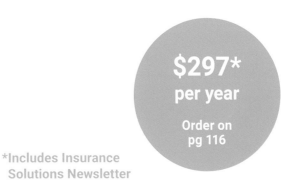

$297* **per year**

Order on pg 116

***Includes Insurance Solutions Newsletter**

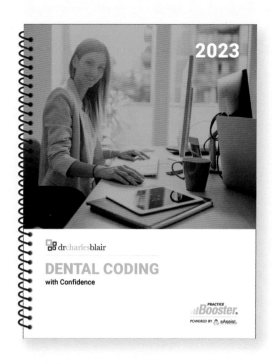

THE "GO TO" DENTAL CODING GUIDE

Dental Coding With Confidence is dentistry's premier CDT coding guide. Exclusive reader-friendly graphics arm your dental team with the ability to prevent the most common and costly coding errors. Plus, comprehensive content includes expert comments about each code, dental plan limitations, and key narrative guidance needed to successfully submit dental claims to gain maximum and timely reimbursement. This is a must-have for your dental practice! Ensure correct coding with the *CDT 2023 Edition of Dental Coding With Confidence.*

Order your copy of the **2023 Dental Coding With Confidence** today!

Order form on page 116

Order form on page 116

Dental Coding With Confidence

TOP REASONS this Guide is a must-have for your practice:

- Stay up-to-date with the 2023 annual additions, revisions, and deletions to dentistry's CDT codes

- Proven PREDICTIVE ERROR CORRECTION® helps predict common errors before you make them

- Understand proper dental coding and learn insurance claim submission tips to maximize legitimate reimbursement

- Know when and how to properly report current 2023 CDT codes

CDT 2023 Updates:

- 22 New Codes
- 14 Revised Codes
- 0 Editorial Revisions
- 2 Deleted Codes

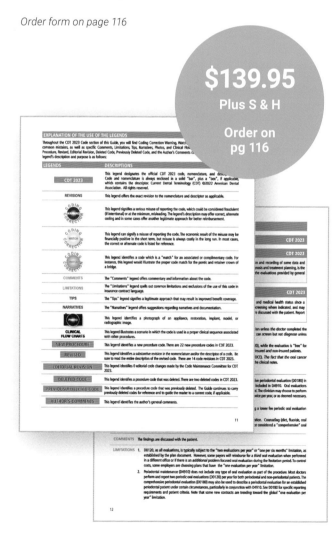

$139.95
Plus S & H

Order on
pg 116

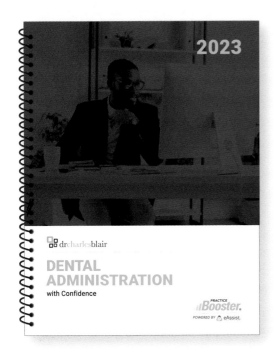

Empower your dental team with critical need-to-know information to successfully navigate the hurdles of everyday dental insurance administration.

This guide is filled with proven solutions for both common and complex problems facing every practice today. Dental Administration With Confidence is easy to understand and packed full with information, tools, and solutions to help your team maximize reimbursement, reduce claim denials and delays, increase patient satisfaction, and boost revenue. Plus, it is perfect for both the new and experienced team member!

Order your copy of the **2023 Dental Administration With Confidence** today!

Order form on page 116

Dental Administration With Confidence

Features and Content:

- Maximizing legitimate reimbursement

- Details on plan types – (PPOs, DHMOs, Federal/State, etc.)

- Coordination of benefits – properly calculating patient responsibility and adjustments

- Frequently asked administrative and coding Q&As

- Sample checklists, patient and financial forms, and letters

- Exclusive access to online bonus content and more!

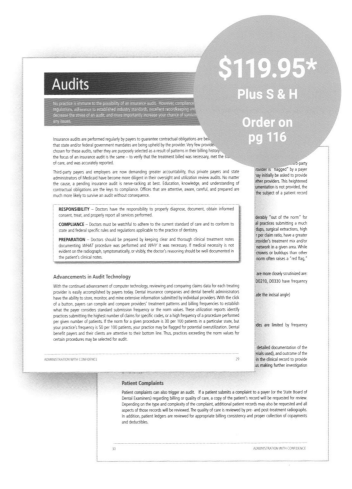

$119.95*
Plus S & H

Order on pg 116

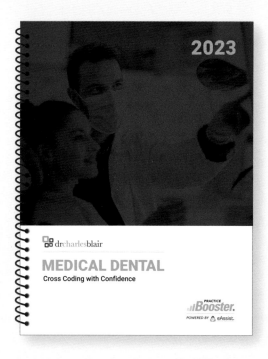

Medical Dental Cross Coding With Confidence

Features and New Content for 2023

- Evaluation and Management Guidelines for 2023

- Cross Coding CDT to CPT® Procedure Codes (includes new 2023 CDT codes)

- Expert Billing Tips Included on Each Coding Page

- Medicare and Medicare Advantage Plan Information for the Dental Practice

- How to Successfully Submit Claims to Medical Payors for Dental-Related Trauma, Surgical Extractions, Third Molar Extractions, TMJ, GERD, Sleep Apnea and More

- Instructions on How to Complete the CMS 1500 (02-12) Medical Claim Form

- Clinical Scenarios with Examples of Completed Medical Claim Forms

- How to Report ICD-10-CM Diagnoses Codes on Medical and Dental Claims

- Exclusive On-Line Access to Bonus Information and Updates

Medical Dental Cross Coding With Confidence empowers dental teams to conquer the complexities of medical claim submission for dental practices. Learn from easy-to-follow clinical scenarios and receive step-by-step instructions for completing the CMS 1500 (02-12) Medical Claim Form.

More dental plans are increasingly mandating the submission of certain procedures (such as surgical extractions, bone grafting, etc.) along with procedures considered medical in nature (such as biopsies, dental trauma, TMD treatments, sleep apnea appliances, etc.) to the patient's medical plan before submission to the patient's dental plan. Due to this trend, dental teams are now faced with the task of filing procedures to the patient's medical plan more often, but many teams struggle.

No matter your experience level, this is a must-have for every practice! This exceptional resource explains the different types of medical codes, how to complete the medical claim form, and how to submit proper claims to medical payors. Additionally, this Manual explains how to properly apply ICD-10-CM codes to the dental claim form using the Scenario Based Teaching Method℠. Eliminate the apprehension of filing medical claims in your practice with the straightforward guidance in this indispensable manual!

Order your copy of the *2023 Medical Dental Cross Coding With Confidence* today to learn how to successfully submit medical claims for various dental procedures, including surgical extractions, dental related trauma, accidents, sleep apnea, TMJ, and much more!

Order form on page 116

$349.95
Plus S & H

Order on pg 116

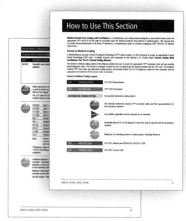

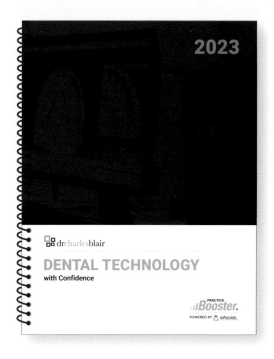

Are you thinking about purchasing that 3D Printer or Laser on your wish list? Considering placing and/or restoring Implants? Whether you are a specialist or a general dentist that specializes in innovative procedures, **Dental Technology With Confidence** provides insurance coding and administration insight on the technological advancements in dentistry. Incorporating state of the art technology into your practice or expanding your skill set can elevate the quality of care you provide your patients. With Dental Technology With Confidence at your fingertips, you can feel confident in navigating the confusing world of insurance as it relates to these advancements..

No matter your experience level, this is a must-have for every practice! This exceptional resource will help you prevent common errors and maximize legitimate reimbursement for forward thinking practices.

Order your copy of the **2023 Dental Technology With Confidence** today!

Order form on page 116

Dental Technology With Confidence

Features and Content:

- Tips and tricks on dental & medical coding for CBCT

- Learn how to document for CAD/CAM

- Eliminate the confusion of implants

- Learn how to implement lab testing into your practice

- Discover how to get the most out of your laser

- Uncover dental and medical coding for sleep dentistry

- Learn how to get paid through medical insurance for TMD

- Learn the many ways you can use 3D printing in your practice

- Discover more about stationary tomosynthesis and how it will revolutionize the way you take radiographs

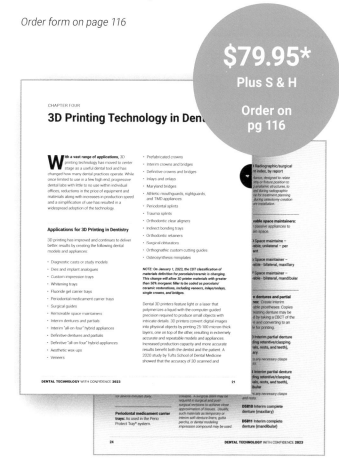

$79.95*
Plus S & H

Order on pg 116

Order form

○ **Dental Coding With Confidence** / **$139.95* + $10 S/H**

○ **Dental Administration With Confidence** / **$119.95* + $10 S/H**

○ **Bundle (Coding and Administration With Confidence)** / **$229.95* + $15 S/H**

○ **Medical Dental Cross Coding With Confidence** / **$349.95* + $20 S/H**

○ **Dental Technology With Confidence** / **$79.95* + $10 S/H**

○ **Practice Booster** / **$297 per year** (Includes Insurance Solutions Newsletter)

Plus applicable sales tax for NC only

PRACTICE INFORMATION

Practice Name:

Attn:

Address:

City: State: Zip:

Telephone: Email:

Order Online: www.practicebooster.com/store

Mail to: Practice Booster, P.O. Box 986, Belmont, NC 28012-0986

Fax to: 704.825.3960

METHOD OF PAYMENT

○ Check # *(Payable to Practice Booster):*   Amount:

○ Visa   ○ Mastercard   ○ AMEX   ○ Discover

Card #:

Exp. Date: /   Security #:

Signature

P.O. Box 986 Belmont, NC 28012-0986
Phone: 704.829.3194
Fax: 704.825.3960
www.practicebooster.com
email: info@practicebooster.com

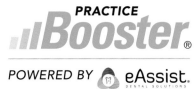

CONSULTING SERVICES

Revenue Enhancement Program

Is your practice losing hundreds of dollars every single day due to lack of current CDT knowledge, improper fee positioning, and clinical protocols?

If you're not maintaining a balanced fee schedule, implementing up-to-date clinical procedure protocols and using the latest insurance code set, it could cost you tens of thousands of dollars in unrealized profit this year alone.

Don't gamble with the financial health of your practice. Take the guesswork out of fees and treatment protocols with the Revenue Enhancement Program.

The Revenue Enhancement Program utilizes Predictive Error Correction.

___

Program highlights

- **2½ – 3- hour telephone consultation for the doctor and staff** to analyze your insurance coding, clinical protocols, procedure utilization rates, and scope of services with specific recommendations for improvement.

- **Information on any new insurance coding,** interpretations, and insurance updates.

- **Includes a 1-year subscription to our online Practice Booster® Code Advisor,** a powerful search engine for dental coding and billing, along with sample narratives, pertinent coding articles by Insurance Solutions Newsletter, and much more.

- **Complimentary copy of Dr. Blair's manual,** *Dental Administration With Confidence: The "Go To" Guide For Insurance Administration.*

- **One year of follow-up support** with answers to you and your team's questions on insurance and proper coding.

- **Fee schedule rebalancing.**

Take the guesswork out of correct coding and reimbursement, setting fees, and PPO feasibility/analysis.

> "
> Dr. Blair's Revenue Enhancement Program was a vital part of my practice's success. Because of his well thought out advice, thorough review of our revenue sources, counsel regarding our coding, and his ongoing availability, I was able to sell my practice at age 55 and move on to a fruitful second career: I graduated from seminary (debt free!), was ordained, and now serve joyfully in my church. I urge all the dentists out there to work with Dr. Blair in achieving their practice goals ethically and efficiently."
>
> — RAD ORLANDI, DDS

For more information, please email Julie Devinney at julie@practicebooster.com or visit https://www.practicebooster.com/revenue-enhancement.asp

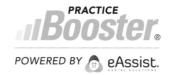

PRACTICE
ıllBooster. ®

POWERED BY ▲ eAssist.

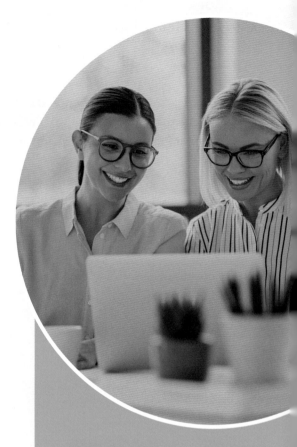
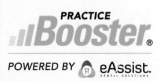